Excuse Me!
Is This Your Body?

Excuse Me!
Is This Your Body?

Abbas Ghadimi

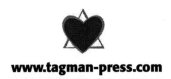

www.tagman-press.com

First published in July 2006 by Tagman Worldwide Ltd in
The Tagman Press Crown Laurel imprint

Tagman Worldwide Ltd
Lovemore House, PO Box 754, Norwich NR1 4GY England UK
Tel: 0845 644 4186
Fax: 0845 644 4187
www.tagman-press.com
Email: editorial@tagman-press.com

© Copyright (text and front cover image) 2006 by Abbas Ghadimi

The right of Abbas Ghadimi to be identified as the author of this work has been asserted by him in accordance with the Copyright, Designs & Patents Act 1988.

All rights reserved. No part of this publication may be reproduced, stored in a retrieval system or transmitted in any form or by any means, electronic, mechanical, recording or otherwise, without the prior written permission of the authors and copyright holders.

ISBN – Paperback 1-903571-60-X

A CIP catalogue record for this book is available from the British Library

Cover Design and Illustrations: Kevin Jones

Text Design and Printing by CLE Print Ltd, St Ives, Cambridgeshire

CONTENTS

Foreword by Anthony Grey i

My Dream vi

Author's Introduction viii

The Four Golden Principles xiii

Chapter One   How This Book Was Born 1

Chapter Two   My Life and the Subject of Health 8

Chapter Three   Telling Stories and Writing Books 14

Chapter Four   Where Does It All Begin? 22

Chapter Five   The Process of Digestion 34

Chapter Six   Illness and Wellness – the Connections 47

Chapter Seven   Wellness – How I Love that Term! 75

Chapter Eight   Principle No 1 – Be Grateful 79

Chapter Nine   Principle No 2 – Drink Enough Water 91

Chapter Ten   Principle No 3 – Eat Less and Move More ... 100

Chapter Eleven   Principle No 4 – Nutrition 131

Chapter Twelve   Heart to Heart 175

Appendix   Great Healers, Past and Present 183

Acknowledgements 188

Contact Information 189

*This book is dedicated to my very dear wife Carmel Rose
for her unwavering love, support and assistance
that made it all possible*

FOREWORD

by Anthony Grey

Excuse Me – Is This Your Body? is one of the most remarkable health books I have ever read. It is written in an idiosyncratic and light-hearted style which begins right at the start with its engaging title and the author's highly original cover images of gold ingots, diamonds and bank notes planted provocatively in our major bodily organs to shake us into thinking in new ways about our bodies and how we value and treat them. Then it moves immediately to braid together diverse strands of positive information about health and wellness from vastly different cultural and scientific sources that are all potentially life-changing.

The sources, uniquely in my view, bridge a number of disparate disciplines from the East and the West, which normally remain separate, ignored or unreconciled in our deeply troubled modern world.

The philosophical and medical wisdom of the ancient Persian and Grecian cultures is blended with canny Persian folklore remedies, mainstream Western medical science, German-inspired homeopathy and an everyday, commonsense intuitive approach to health and wellbeing. All are skilfully combined to produce a simple, easily understood body of irresistible advice that urges the reader to take full responsibility immediately for his or her own health by applying a few simple rules about mental attitudes towards our eating and drinking habits, our exercise regimes, and our food knowledge.

The common denominator for the drawing together of these diverse strands is the knowledge, life experience and ebullient personality of the author, Abbas Ghadimi. An engaging, Iranian-born, Ireland-based practitioner of many linked complementary healthcare arts, Abbas writes mostly in a spoken vernacular, addressing his readers with intimate familiarity like an ancient Persian village soothsayer seated before an evening campfire with a circle of intent and enthralled listeners hanging on his every word.

At other times he observes, analyses and blends in the scientific findings of Western medical research. He also draws on nearly twenty years of experience in healthcare roles at different levels in Ireland – first as a grower and seller door-to-door of organic vegetables, then as a health food storeowner and eventually a full-time homeopathic practitioner.

All these unlikely strands came to be woven together in Ireland because Abbas chose to move there in 1985 following a desperate night time flight by truck out of Iran. He crossed a desolate desert to land up in a refugee camp in Pakistan in the wake of the overthrow of Shah Pahlavi.

At the core of this work Abbas spells out very simply four fundamental golden principles, which, he is confident, will bring about improved health and wellbeing for anyone and everyone who takes the time to practice them diligently. They are in brief : First: BE GRATEFUL and think primarily always of what is right in your life before anything else. Second: DRINK ENOUGH WATER. Third: EAT LESS AND MOVE MORE. Fourth: NUTRITION – study and apply a few important elementary rules which can be summed up under the simple heading: *Let food be your medicine and medicine be your food.*

These four golden principles, says Abbas, are synthesised from the combined wisdom of the ages mixed with modern medical science and the best complementary health care principles. They are spelled out in detail in their own separate chapters towards the end of the book – and like the rest of this lively narrative, are interspersed with entertaining and meaningful anecdotes from ancient and modern sources that together memorably punch home the author's points with great force. I defy anybody who truly cares about their health to read about these four principles and their application and not feel moved to implement at least some of them immediately. As I read through the first draft manuscript of the book, I began modifying my own ways of daily living to embody a lot of these ideas!

I will here select just one powerful example of the sort of information it contains. At one point Abbas describes how new scientific research has proved that thoughts that come under Golden Principle No 1 – Be Grateful, actually stimulate the direct and instant secretion of beneficial hormones or neurotransmitters such as Dopamine in our bodies that otherwise would not be produced. Serotonin and Melatonin can also be stimulated by similar positive thoughts and feelings. What an extraordinary encouragement to practice and apply that first Golden Principle immediately on waking each day!

The rest of this kaleidoscope of considered wisdom I will leave you to discover gradually for yourselves as you journey through a charming landscape of facts, figures and passionate exhortations. What I would just like to emphasise is that the author is totally convincing when he says that all he truly wishes to do is to reach out and touch your heart with these beneficial insights which he has proved to be true during nearly twenty years of treating clients and studying and researching his subject in all directions.

There is another remarkable connection between myself, The Tagman Press and Abbas Ghadimi that must be revealed here. For six years Tagman, which I founded in the late 1990s has published a series of groundbreaking and revolutionary health books by another Iranian-born author Dr Fereydoon Batmanghelidj who wrote the phenomenal worldwide bestseller *Your Body's Many Cries for Water* which has sold over a million copies in the United States and other countries and some 60,000 copies in the United Kingdom in recent years.

Dr Batmanghelidj, who died in 2004, has affectionately become known as 'Dr Batman' or 'Dr B' by millions of his readers and I first met Abbas when I telephoned him cold in Kilkenny to see who it was with such an exotic non-Irish name that was ordering so many of Dr B's books through the Tagman website. In fact I found he was giving the books away or selling them onward at health talks by himself because of their importance. So the Second Golden Principle of this book – Drink Enough Water – is firmly based around the extraordinary lexicon of work produced by Dr Batmanghelidj, who made his ground-breaking discoveries whilst under sentence of death in a Teheran prison following the 1979 revolution in Iran.

Yet in this new book Abbas also consciously adds to and augments Dr B's work in writing about both the Second Golden Principle and indeed with the whole spectrum of his own broader advice contained in these pages. In a very real sense Dr B's mission is being admiringly continued and extended by his younger fellow countryman Abbas Ghadimi – as well as by The Tagman Press and myself.

Yet this book is not just an end in itself. It is also the starting point and a major part of a larger ambition which Abbas himself describes on the next two pages under the simple heading 'My Dream.' While setting out details of comprehensive new methods by means of which we can help ourselves achieve optimum health and wellbeing, he simultaneously points out what is seriously wrong with our conventional mainstream healthcare systems. In effect he is practising a prophetic vocation by foretelling the new, while courageously challenging the old.

To counteract and correct the situation, Abbas envisages creating a new and revolutionary way of dealing with health matters in society by shifting the exclusive focus away from hospitals that so evidently treat the already sick and injured. He plans to do this by creating first in Ireland and later all over the world, what he terms Wellness Homes. In such centres the philosophy and methods advocated by this book will be put into practice and in such settings people will be helped gently to understand how to sustain or regain their good health by applying these positive principles.

By his rare skills, deep knowledge and his passionate dedication to restoring and sustaining good health, Abbas Ghadimi has already helped thousands of people in the Republic of Ireland over the past two decades to find their way to new levels of wellbeing and happiness. This book is a landmark, I am sure, in that continuing journey of dedication to healthcare of the broadest kind – and I feel sure it marks a point where those numbers are now going to swell into tens of thousands and possibly hundreds of thousands and more via publication of this book and Abbas's growing number of public talks and his plans to found the Wellness Homes in Ireland and beyond.

Lastly and perhaps most importantly, the positive bridges this book uniquely builds between Eastern cultures and Western society carry in my opinion, a deeper symbolic and practical significance. While dealing directly with peaceful and positive health matters this narrative also helps convey in a new and refreshing way how much can be gained if we direct our caring and compassionate attention to what joins, benefits and unites us in our past and present cultures rather than what so much more easily can divide, harm and destroy.

It is also a fine example of how the trauma and setback of being forced to flee your own country for political reasons and live in exile abroad – as Dr Batmanghelidj also did – can be overcome to bring change and greater benefit to the world. Dr Batmanghelidj and Abbas Ghadimi are together and separately remarkable representatives of their native country and its cultural richness and diversity that often seems to be overlooked today. For their contributions in the West to our understanding of our own health and how to enhance and sustain it, both authors in my view deserve our sincerest congratulations and warmest thanks.

Anthony Grey,
Spring 2006, Norwich, England

Anthony Grey is a former foreign correspondent with Reuters news agency in Berlin, Eastern Europe and China. After being held hostage for two years by Red Guards in China he worked as a BBC World Service radio and television broadcaster. He is perhaps best known as the author of the international best selling historical novels, SAIGON, PEKING, THE BANGKOK SECRET and TOKYO BAY. He is also chairman and founder of The Tagman Press publishing imprint.

MY DREAM

Like many people I have a dream – and I will do whatever it takes to achieve my dream.

The seed of my dream was sown in me when I was seven years old. My Grandma became very ill after a favourite uncle of hers died. The illness was very sudden and the doctors had no idea what it was. She lay in bed without talking and ate very little for a whole month. My Grandpa was very distraught until somebody suggested to him that he call in a special doctor who was known locally as the **'ONE PRESCRIPTION DOCTOR'** His name was **DR. FARHANGY**.

When he came to see my granny, Dr Farhangy made a great impression on me. He always said to me: 'How is my little friend today?' His methods of healing were simple and very effective. He looked at the whole situation of the person and not just the symptoms. My Granny's prescription was to have one sweet melon each day and he suggested we get a fan for her because the heat was so intense in the summer months in Persia.

We could not afford to buy a fan at that time so he gave us one from his office and with these simple remedies she quickly recovered.. The kindness of this man impressed me so much that I decided there and then I would be a great doctor one day just like Dr Farhangy.

Then time moved on and I put my dream away like most young children do. I got on with my life, which took many twists and turns. Then one day after I left Iran to live in Ireland, my interest in health through homeopathy rekindled my childhood dream. Memories of that time emerged suddenly from deep within me and I remembered the great Dr Farhangy again and my promises to myself to be like him.

The ancient Persian physician **Abu Alie Cinna** once said:

THE GOAL OF MEDICINE MUST BE TO FOCUS ON PROTECTING HEALTH DURING PERIODS OF WELLBEING AND RESTORING HEALTH IN PERIODS OF ILLNESS.

So inspired by this ancient saying and Dr Farhangy's example, this is what my dream has become: to build a **WELLNESS HOME** or a series of Wellness Homes to help people to focus on their own wellbeing, to teach them how to stay well, how to see the specialness of their lives and their health, to have a place where they can come to stay healthy, to get healthy if they are ill, to recover after illness.

Whatever an individual's needs are, these Wellness Homes will be able to help them. The homes can work in conjunction with hospitals because we need hospitals and their staff to be free for when they are most needed – for emergencies, operations and accidents. Our hospitals are filled with people who could be well with only small adjustments to their lifestyle. Above all else we need to take responsibility for our own health and wellbeing.

These Wellness Homes will teach people how to do just that. However, such homes will not come into being unless we all contribute to their existence. They need everybody's input. So if you feel you have something to contribute to this new way of becoming healthy and staying healthy and would like to participate, I have added contact information for myself at the back of this book.

For my part for now, I will say, as long as I can take breath in this wonderful gift of life I will pursue *my dream*. For whether we realise it or not, our health is the ultimate gift of abundance.

Abbas Ghadimi
Kilkenny, Ireland, Spring 2006

AUTHOR'S INTRODUCTION

The title of this book is *Excuse Me! Is This Your Body?* and the imaginary picture I devised for its cover shows items of wealth stored away inside us to emphasise the supreme importance of the wellbeing of all our internal organs. To make the point strongly they are compared to exchangeable valuables such as money, gold, diamonds and jewellery in general which we value so highly in our everyday material lives

Let's begin with the **BRAIN**, which is a part of our central nervous system and is in charge of many functions, amongst them the control of sleep, thirst, hunger and sexual desires. The purpose of the gold bars seen in the head is to bring to our attention that the brain is like a **GOLD MINE** and needs to be treated as a very precious commodity. We know a gold mine also contains many other things besides gold, like dust, sand and stone, so those things need to be separated out. Our brain also contains lots of undesirable thoughts as well as many golden thoughts such as dreams, goals, our concern for others, our desires to love or to be loved and to serve mankind. As you can imagine these golden thoughts do not always come easily to us; we all need to work harder like miners to dig out and find the hidden gold in all our minds – and this book tells us how.

The next organs we need to look at are our **LUNGS**, which provide the oxygen to our body and release the carbon dioxide. Oxygen is the first and most important substance for survival of any living thing so ensuring a proper supply of oxygen to our body is as important or more important even than having a savings account. It is as if we are day by day depositing money to that vital account and if we do not supply the body properly with sufficient oxygen via our lungs and load it instead with a lot of carbon dioxide, it is like withdrawing money all the time from that vital account, our lungs. If that happens we may 'bankrupt' our physical system and it will shut down.

The next organs we need to look at are our **LIVER** and **GALLBLADDER**. Our liver is like a large chemical factory and our gallbladder can be seen as a jewellery shop.

As we know in a jewellery shop one can find all kinds of jewellery. In fact jewellery is concentrated wealth and so is our liver and gallbladder. Large amounts of concentrated wealth like gallstones can sometimes be found there which are concentrated fat mixed with bile and some calcium. Actually gallstones mostly are fat; in other words if we put gallstones into a frying pan they dissolve.

In our daily life if we are in a financial crisis we can exchange our jewellery against other currencies in order to survive. Similarly the gallstone also can be exchanged for a supply of energy for a while and we need to know that gallstones can be eliminated by blending a combination of **OLIVE OIL, APPLE JUICE, FRESH OR GROUND GINGER, LEMON JUICE** and some **CAYENNE PEPPER**. This can also be achieved by fasting for many days with water alone. But please, please, please, do not apply this recommendation without consulting a competent physician if you suffer from gallstones or you are easily prone to gallstones.

It is exactly the same with the liver. Our liver contains and stores all kinds of chemicals and fat and bile which can be seen to function in the same way as jewellery in our economy.

Other important organs that we need to focus on are our **ORGANS OF ELIMINATION** which as their name indicates are concerned solely with movement and eliminating matter. That is why I have placed a lot of coins in this area which we call '**CHANGE**' or '**SMALL CHANGE**'. In order to have a healthy body we need to have regular bowel movements or in other words we need to change the contents of the elimination organs daily. Many natural physicians believe that death starts from the colon – or it is better said that death starts from **BLOCKAGE** of the colon.

In this connection I remember some time back hearing a story about a king in Persia who had a desire for his daughter to marry. He announced that any man who considered himself to be a wise man could come forward and convince him of his ability and wisdom. He would then be prepared happily to give his daughter to him. But if the claimants failed to prove their ability, he would put them in prison. In this way, he thought, he could eliminate many undesirable inquires.

Day by day many people came to the palace to offer wisdom but not enough to convince the king. Soon the prison was almost full of people, until one day, a particular young man came to the palace smiling and offered this wisdom to the king.

'Dear King.' he said, 'I feel that you should let me marry your daughter, since I am not only the wisest man in this land but also the luckiest person too. The reason for this is I am able to have a good bowel movement everyday.'

The King not only was surprised but even became angry with this seemingly foolish statement and immediately ordered his guards to put the young man in prison.

But the young man still smiled and bowed saying: 'My lord I am still the luckiest man of this land even if you put me in prison. You can find this out for yourself. Try to ignore your bowel activity and you will see for yourself that you are not able to last for very long.'

That same night when the king was in bed he found himself thinking about the young man. He decided to ignore the activity of his bowel movement and see what would happen. For a day or two he was able to handle the challenge but by the third or fourth day the pressure was so strong that he had to go to the bathroom and give up his contributions for the betterment of the environment. During and shortly after the performance he found himself saying:

"THANKS BE TO GOD THAT I CAN DO THIS – I AM TRULY A LUCKY MAN"

Then he immediately remembered the young man in prison and ordered his guards to release him at once so that he could fulfil his promise to allow him marry his daughter.

When the young man was free he said to the King: 'I will marry your daughter – but only if you free all the other people who are in prison for seeking her hand.'

This statement instantly brought a satisfied smile to the king's face. Inside his head he heard a voice saying:

"HE IS NOT ONLY A WISE MAN, BUT ALSO HE IS A KIND MAN"

Then the King and the princess and her husband and the people in the kingdom all lived happily ever after, going regularly to the bathroom every day, presenting their contributions back to the environment.

* * * * * * * * *

I have left until last the most important organ of all in our bodies – our **HEART**. For the **HEART** is not only an organ, but rather the centre of our whole being. Although the heart is in a person's body in the chest cavity it is equally true, I feel, that each person is equally in their own heart. In other words:

"YOUR HEART IS IN YOU AND YOU ARE IN YOUR HEART"

Without **HEART**, a person is dead and there is no life force.

Equally in society and in every country in the world the **TREASURY** is the control centre of the economy. I have represented that on the cover of this book by a symbolic **TREASURE CHEST** containing all the different forms of money, gold, silver, jewels and all kinds of valuables. Each country's economy is backed up by gold or diamonds or labour and technology and these effectively become the spirit or soul of the country. And it is just the same with the heart.

The soul or spirit of the person is in the heart, we fall in love with our heart we feel hurt with our **HEART** because the memory of the joy or hurt remains in the heart. Our **HEART** keeps the memory of our life. Every minute of every day of our lives is stored in our heart. When a person's HEART has so much hurt in it, that person finds it hard to trust others. That is why there is a great phrase which says:

"IF YOU'RE FEELING HURT, LET THE INJURY GO AND YOU WILL BE FREE"

In other words **FORGIVE AND FORGET**!

Our HEART is more than an organ; it is indeed our greatest **TREASURE**, our **TREASURE CHEST** because it is all of our being – as

I point out in the final concluding section of this book, Chapter 12 which is entitled **HEART TO HEART**. There I refer to the heart being 'the seat of God's throne.'

There is no currency which can describe the **HEART** since the **HEART** is as I have said, the **TREASURY** and currency takes its meaning or value from it. The most common currency in the world is paper money which merely is paper bearing pictures that are backed up by the **TREASURY** of the country in order to give it value. In essence such money is only paper.

The economy of our body is dependent on our **HEART** in the same way that the economy of a country is dependent on its **TREASURY**. The only good reason for reading and applying the contents of this book in your life is if it makes you feel good in your **HEART**. If you merely enjoy it but do not apply its teachings, you will not benefit from it in the long term.

Therefore I wish and I hope and I pray that the contents of this book will touch your **HEART** enough for you to take action. Then the efforts of all involved in its production will have been worthwhile. All I am saying to you realy is:

EXCUSE ME! IS THIS YOUR BODY?

THE FOUR GOLDEN PRINCIPLES OF GOOD HEALTH AND WELLBEING

At the core of this book, spelled out in detail in Chapters Eight, Nine, Ten and Eleven are four essential 'golden' principles for building and maintaining good health and wellbeing. To help you start thinking about them straight away they are listed briefly here:

1 BE GRATEFUL – ALWAYS THINK FIRST WHAT IS RIGHT IN YOUR LIFE

2 DRINK ENOUGH WATER – YOU'RE NOT SICK YOU'RE THIRSTY!

3 EAT LESS AND MOVE MORE – JUST DO IT!

4 NUTRITION – LET FOOD BE YOUR MEDICINE AND MEDICINE BE YOUR FOOD

CHAPTER ONE

HOW THIS BOOK WAS BORN

'Why don't you write a book?'

It is almost 15 years ago since I was asked that question by one of my weekly customers in a health food store that I owned at that time.

'Me?' I asked.

'Yes, you,' he replied.

'What do I have to say that hasn't been said before,' I asked. 'Or is so important that I should write a book on it?'

My customer said; 'Well in my opinion you know things about health and wellness which is unique and comprehensive. Besides the most important thing is this: you have a way of simplifying the complexities of health and disease.'

That's how the seed of having a desire to write a book was sown in me at that time – and now at last it is bearing fruit.

The reason this man's question made me think of writing a book was because of his character and I will try my best to describe him to you.

He was around fifty years old and always wore very, very, ragged clothes. His hair was light and long and he always carried a rucksack known in the area as a Czech bag, (a bag made in the Czech Republic). He was a driver for one of the local organisations and on his day off each week he would drop in for his shopping and our little chat.

But most important of all he seemed to know something about almost everything. He told me he had read at least one or two books a week for 25 years. He knew about herbs, plants, politics, geography, places and peoples: you name it he knew something about it.

When one would see him in the street one would not believe how knowledgeable a person he was. Yet we had weekly conversations, about all sorts of things – and mostly about new discoveries in the health area.

Now I know how much I miss our weekly conversations, **GOD BLESS HIM** !

So the dream of writing a book was buried in me for many years. Then a few years ago my wife asked me the same question: 'Why don't you write a book?'

Again I thought about it. But I did nothing until in 2005 she said it again. And this time it was: 'You really should seriously think about writing a book!'

So here it is; and I hope you enjoy reading it as much as I have enjoyed writing it.

* * * * * * * * *

I would like to say first that this book is written specially for you, dear reader and that your health and wellbeing is the main purpose for it. In fact that is the sole reason why it has come into existence.

I would like you to know that, there were hundreds or even thousands of aware doctors, ancient physicians, modern scientists, and other invisible beings that were called upon in order to get this book written and get it to your hands. No matter where you are reading it right now, sitting on a bus or a train or an aeroplane or the smallest room in your house (I will leave that to your imagination), perhaps you have been given this book as a present or you have just picked it up in a book store – whichever it was, or perhaps synchronised universal circumstances have put this book into your hands.

As a result, from now on you have become responsible for the achievement of optimal **HEALTH** for your body. When you take responsibility for your **HEALTH** you gain power from this choice, rather than giving that power away.

What you do with this choice is entirely up to you.

You can just drop it, and forget you have ever seen it.

Or you can just have faith and follow and fulfil the most joyful act of your life.

How This Book Was Born

You may ask: Why should I bother?   What is in it for me?

The answers to those questions are: **Because you need your health.**

If you only knew what I know!! I promise you that when you read this information and totally apply it in your life, and when it works for you, suggest it to your nearest and dearest; the following rewards could be yours.

1. As far as I am aware, you will have the possibility of gaining not only your greatest asset, but the only one of really lasting value – that is **YOUR HEALTH.**

2. You will have the possibility of seeing your nearest and dearest ones become **WELL** and **FREE** from the long term and unnecessary misery of ill health in which you may have heard the words: 'Sorry, that is all we can do!

3. In other words you can be rewarded by seeing them avoid the misery of hospitalisation.

4. And finally, by the will of the Creator we will all experience half full or even empty hospitals and more healthy people in this big noisy world of humanity.

Overall it is clear that **HEALTH** does not come about by academic knowledge, neither by learning from books or attending a variety of seminars and conferences, or going through routine check ups, or following a specific diet.

HEALTH is freedom and movement, **HEALTH** is the ability to cope with our environment, **MENTALLY, EMOTIONALLY** and **PHYSICALLY,** and can only be achieved by applying the knowledge that we have learned.

No one can learn how to swim by reading books, we can only learn by jumping into the water, and practising what we have learned.

In my opinion, only one thing can bring about a passion for health and that is an **EMOTIONAL ATTACHMENT** to the outcome or a strong desire to be healthy and nothing else can equalise this power.

I heard a beautiful quote from **Mother Teresa of Calcutta** which says:

"UNLESS THERE IS A WILLINGNESS TO HEAL, THE DISEASE CAN NOT BE BEATEN"

The driving force of illness is **FEAR;** the driving force of health is **LOVE.**

Today medical systems focus on **ILL CARE** not **HEALTH CARE.**

As one quote I heard said, 'We have an overwhelming, wasteful, expensive, frightening, and inhuman medical system.'

I know you may say this is a huge statement and hard to believe.

Our doctors and nurses work in their profession with the love of their patients in their hearts, there is no doubt about that, but the system does not allow them the time they need to implement the care they may wish, because of the overwhelming pressure imposed on them.

Look, what have you got to lose?

I don't know, possibly these may be some of the things that you could lose.

A   Maybe you will lose that never ending pain that you always had.

B   Or lose that extra weight which bothers you.

C   Or priceless time that you spend in a waiting room of some physician, that in their best capability can only offer you a pain killer?

Well just at least read it. When you finish, you will have 4 principles, to follow, which can be written on the back of a business card, and so easy to apply that no one can make it complicated, unless they are a genius.

Please realise that you are in the driver's seat.

This is the only 'have to' you need to follow; the rest will come to you very easily.

You need to know that you are the owner of your body; you are in charge of it. I am not sure this is good news for you or bad news!!

If you take care of your wellbeing it is good news, but if you abuse your body then it is not good news.

How This Book Was Born

You need to know that it is **YOU** who are responsible for your wellbeing, no one else, and you need to take care of it.

Besides, if you don't take care of your body, and end up with a dilapidated one, where else are you going to live?

It is you who makes the choice.

It is you who goes to the same physician, either medical doctor or alternative physician, for many years without having a satisfying result, but still keep going back to them.

I have been so privileged to work with thousands of people.

One thing, and only one thing, that I strongly can make a statement about is the action and willingness of a person who wants to get well, can bring about health and optimum wellbeing. No other tool can be as close as this simple thing, which can take us off of the merry-go-round, of the complexity of ill health.

As I write this I am wishing very strongly that you will hear and understand me. I wish also that you be able to see and understand what I can see and have seen.

As I see it my responsibility is to get this information to you; from here the rest is all up to you.

All I can say is good luck, and have patience with yourself.

I am going to do my best to give to you what I observed and learned from dealing with thousands of people whom I have treated, and also I will give you the essence of the learning that I have from ancient Persian and Arabic books combined with modern science of the western world, in a simple and applicable principle for you.

So these are the foods which have been prepared for you to receive, I hope you enjoy them.

Finally, I would like to give you a picture that hopefully can bring about an emotional connection between you and your body.

Imagine you are watching a movie, and it is about parents who have a lot of children in the house to feed. But they do not bother to feed the children proper foods, so the children scream with the pain of hunger and malnutrition, and their parents carelessly spend the money on drink, cigarettes and other stimulant substances.

How would you feel about people like that ?

I know I would feel disheartened for the children; in fact such parents can be brought before the courts for cruelty and child abuse. Now you tell me what is the difference between not feeding those children and the cells and tissues and organs in our bodies? They are in your hands to be well fed and looked after properly. Your body is your home you need to take care of it.

I wish you all the best and you can be assured of my prayers for your success. Believe me:

YOU CAN DO IT!

I prefer a short life
with
WIDTH
to a narrow one
with
LENGTH

*Ibn Sina
(Avicenna)*

CHAPTER TWO

MY LIFE AND THE SUBJECT OF HEALTH

I am originally from Persia, a land of poems, history, and passion. Today of course Persia is known officially as Iran and in this book I use both these terms to refer to my country of birth, which formally became Iran in 1935. Generallly because I will be quoting ancient physicians and sages from earlier times I will use the older name where it is most appropriate. Without getting into too much detail, some of my countrymen still refer to their country as Persia and themselves as Persians despite the official change of name and this is my personal preference also.

I was born into a financially poor family, like a high percentage of the Persian people. My mother's birth was under very unusual circumstances which I believe made a big impact on my own childhood. I would like to share these times with you as I feel it directed my destiny to ignite a spark which has since turned to a fire of passion which I now have for health.

My mother's mother was one of several servants who worked in the house of a Persian royal family, an institution similar to the British royal family, in a small village.

My grandmother became pregnant and at the same time the lady of the house was also pregnant. The birth of their babies came within a few hours of each other. But tragedy struck when the lady of the house lost her child in a 'stillborn' birth and my grandmother died during my mother's birth.

As you can see these were very unusual circumstances, and as the lady of the house, who had lost her child, had sore nipples and breasts full of milk, it was suggested to her that she could feed the servant's child who needed to be breast-fed.

In those days in Persia there was no dry or ready milk as is available

My Life and the Subject of Health

today and often some mothers exchanged feeding their children in times of difficulty or the illness of the real mother.

So it came to be that the royal lady of the house gave breast milk to my mother and that rekindled the light of love that had been extinguished with the loss of her own child. Somehow destiny had brought these two together, mother and baby, with a need for each other through their own tragic loss. Through these strange circumstances the royal lady then became my granny which I refer to in this book.

There was a lot of change in Persia at that time; there was war, food shortages and even a change of government and during this time the Persian Royal family lost everything and had to move to the city.

Some years passed and there was a sudden major reform in the way the country was governed. Disturbances began on the 19 August 1953, which became the most historic day in 100 years of Persia's history (28th of Mordad in the Persian calendar). On the night before, the country was so tense because the Parliament decided that the Shah (King) must leave the country and the army would take over.

In the early morning of 19 August, people went out onto the streets shouting 'Death to the Shah'. The Army tried to stop them and thousands of people lost their lives that morning due to the clashes between anti-Shah factions and the Army. Then in the afternoon and evening the Army brought the country under control again and there were now people on the streets saying 'Long live the Shah'. I was born on that historic day!

My father was a policeman. An uneducated and superstitious man, he was frightened and thought that my birth brought bad luck to the country. He was going to throw me in the river but my Granny stopped him and took me away and we went into hiding.

She often told me stories about that day of my birth and how she really began to love me then. She said that she had no milk to give me and both the city and the countryside were in chaos. So for 18 hours from early morning until midnight I did not have any milk. But the strange thing was that I did not cry even once and she often admired me then for my soft and gentle behaviour.

Excuse Me! Is This Your Body?

That bond between me and my granny, or step granny, was forged from the moment of my birth and the greater part of my life was spent in her house. For a whole month my father did not want even to look at me; then everything settled down in the country and he was all right with me again.

As time went on most of my childhood was the normal lifestyle of a typical poor Persian family, wearing poor clothing, living in poor housing conditions and with very little food. However, I was blessed in that my granny allowed me to spend most of the time in her house. That lifestyle still goes on in Persia today.

I feel most people in the Western world would not be able to comprehend the level of poverty that still exists in many other countries. Our home had rooms alongside each other which housed lots of families in each room and they had low level balconies. My parents and seven children lived in one room. My mother would do the cooking, washing and everything that needed to be done for the whole family in that room.

The only consolation for us was there were other families worse off than us.

It may be hard to imagine how that could be possible, but it was so.

Once someone said that Persia is a rich country with large numbers of financially poor people. Yet somehow we managed and I got an education up to the diploma level that is equivalent in Persia to the Western School Leaving Certificate.

Due to the growing persecution of people of the Baha'i faith during the early years of the war with Iraq, I left Persia in 1984; I had to cross the border from Persia to Pakistan. I was in UN-protected refugee camp in Peshawar, for almost 14 months. The camp was a combination of basic houses of three or four rooms and I was placed in a house, which had three bedrooms, sharing with 16 other people. There were eight people in my room.

I arrived later in Ireland as a part of a Refugee Programme and with the help of Irish friends and some government support I took a course on how to start your own business. Within eight months of finishing the course, I started selling fruit and vegetables door to door. Within a year I made some money which enabled me to open a Health Food Store.

It was then I started my studies, taking a correspondence course on holistic healing and herbal medicine. That course gave me enough knowledge to be able to help people who came to my health shop with acute ailments. But whenever I was confronted by chronic diseases I was not sure what to do. So I decided to make a proper study of health. I studied homoeopathy for four years then took one further year of post graduate studies. I was then practising for four years when I decided to study chronic diseases which I did for two more years.

Three years on I took the one-year Homoeopathic Registration Programme. Today I carry insurance and full registration to practice homoeopathy in Ireland or anywhere in Europe. During many years of dealing with people in my health shop and my clinic I have gained lots of valuable knowledge and priceless experience on health and wellness and I am so grateful to be able to share all this with thousands of people.

I feel blessed to be living in Ireland. It is said that there are almost ten times the population of Ireland at present living outside the country claiming to have some kind of connection to Ireland. The Irish people are well known for being a giving race helping many under-developed and disadvantaged peoples in many areas around the world. I feel privileged to have the good fortune to be living here for almost 20 years, and feel a responsibility to share my knowledge and to give something back.

I feel I am in a privileged position where I have access to the ancient Persian healing writings in their original text and also being blessed by having access to knowledge of modern medicine in the western world. You see I do not wish to end up like my Granny who had a wonderful knowledge of healing, through herbs, foods, and wisdom, and it all went with her when she left this physical life.

So I would like here to pass on to you and future generations some of the wisdom of ancient and modern Persian healers and others, like my Granny, who had an ocean of knowledge about food and herbal medicine.

By doing this I feel I can fulfil my mission of helping people stay healthy. So it is now entirely up to you to do what you will with this book. Reading these pages will help you to understand that the health and wellness principles are simple and easy to follow. But it is only by putting them into action that gives you the chance to receive at first hand an unbelievable result.

And finally, if you find that you receive a good result – and I have no doubt that by following the principles in the following chapters you will do so – please pass on this message to your nearest and dearest. It will fill my heart full of joy to know that I may be making a difference in the world of health and wellness.

**The Only Way for You to Have
a Positive Mental Attitude is
to Create It With Your Own Mind**

CHAPTER THREE

TELLING STORIES AND WRITING BOOKS

Frankly I used to think that people who wrote books were very special and unique individuals – people who had no faults, and a lot of knowledge about everything. But as time passed and I read many books myself, I realised this was not the case. In fact I know now that some of the best books are written by ordinary people.

I now realise that writing books can in fact be a form of service to mankind. Imagine how one can reach into the hearts of thousands of people with just a few pages of information that has been gathered in life as experience of a particular profession or expertise gained in a particular field.

Another thing I have learned is that being a writer can be both a humbling and giving experience. Above all, knowledge is universal and it is so greedy if we do not share it with others.

The most important request I can make to you dear reader at this point is to read this book with an open mind, a forgiving attitude, and a compassionate heart since English is not my mother language. Fortunately, for you, I should add, I have received some help with the language and the book's composition!

But having said that I must add that no matter how much knowledge we have, it can never be comprehensive. Realising this reminded me of a story that was once told to me by a friend who is a graduate of a School of Philosophy in Russia. He told it like this:

It was our last day at university and we were all well dressed and awaiting the last short speech by a professor of Philosophy. Then in walked a skinny old man, his arms dangling by his sides. He moved slowly and a few hairs stuck out from his head looking like pieces of tiny wire. He went over to the blackboard and drew a large circle. In the centre of the circle he drew a small dot and pointing to the large circle, he said: 'This represents the universe that we know exists, and the dot in the centre represents the knowledge mankind has about the universe.'

Then after turning to look briefly at the audience, he left the room.

'We were all absolutely stunned,' said my friend.

In quiet moments often I think about this story. Isn't it true that we are like tiny bugs on Mother Earth, which itself is just like a speck of dust in the universe? Our total life of about 100 years, if we live that long, is like a mere second in time in comparison to the life of the universe.

So what is it all about? It appears that we are all running around like headless chickens up to the last day of our life. It is possible that life appears so real to us that we may think we are going to be around for thousands of years. Well I am sorry if I am disappointing you but we are not.

Just a few decades and it will be all over! (If we even get that much time.)

All those precious **'PRESENT MOMENTS'** of daily life have been wasted, for what? The accumulation of material objects, for example a house a car and all other objects.

However, let me tell you another story – although I think I know what you are going to say now! Here we go again! Is it going to be like this on every second page? Is he going to tell us yet another story?

Well, maybe! I *am* called a storyteller by my friends and clients, so just have patience with me and I hope you enjoy this one.

I know! I know what you are going to say now! I am allowed to tell the story only if I promise not to let the horse of my thoughts run away into the desert of my imagination. Okay! Okay! Honest to God! I will try to go only into the nearby fields and meadows instead of going off deep into the distant deserts.

Well of course I don't mean the **DESSERT** that we get lost in metaphorically at the end of a nice meal – but the **DESERT** in which we can get lost if we don't know where we are going. Isn't the English language really interesting? Just add or subtract one letter S, and you can get lost in two totally different places!

Excuse Me! Is This Your Body?

Well, that is just a thought – or a feeble joke! Try to just smile and keep on reading! At last, I am getting there ...

Once upon a time there was a little spider, who found himself in a nice quiet corner. He set up his web site – in the corner of a kitchen (not on the Internet just in case you were wondering) – and started catching some flies, some mosquitoes and even some moths. As time passed he enjoyed his life until one day just after he had eaten well and was having a nice rest, something unexpected happened.

At the time he had his hands under his head and was reading a book... Oh no! Sorry! Spiders don't read books do they? So he just had his hands under his head and was lying down, his left legs bent and his right feet on his left knees...Can you visualise the picture? Good!

So the spider was thinking: 'I am doing really well in life... Every day I get more flies than I can eat. Just the other day I caught a moth which will be delicious food for weeks... I think now might be a good time for me to get married and settle down and have some children ...'

But just as he was enjoying these lovely imagined scenes of himself being married to a beautiful female spider with long legs and long hair... Ooops, I am not sure that spiders have long hair. But they definitely have long legs, don't they? So anyway with such lovely thoughts in his mind he gently fell into a deep sleep... Khoorrrr, pooffe... Khoorrrr...pooffe.

Then suddenly he was awakened by the loud noise of a door banging. And he heard some human voices. So he rubbed his eyes and stretched himself leisurely because you see, by now, he was very used to hearing human voices.

But this time the noise was constant and this made him really worried. He made an effort to listen closely and he found that it was the voice of the lady of the house informing her maid that an important guest was coming to visit and she needed to clean the kitchen, particularly all the corners.

So the maid started to vacuum everywhere, all the floors, corners, everywhere, and of course the corner of the fridge where the spider had his web site. Poor Spider! Before he had a chance to realise what was happening, he was in the vacuum bag and had been taken to the dustbin.

I know what you are going to say: Oh my God! I will never vacuum up spiders any more. Well my dearest that is not the point, the point is this: Is our own life much different to that of the spider's life? Do we get so comfortable at times we think we are going to be here forever?

This story was first beautifully told 800 years ago by Attar, a famous Persian poet and physician. I have just made some tiny adjustments to fit it into our lifestyle of today. Yet the truth behind this story is confirmed again and again. In fact I know many of my friends, patients and business associates who have been so caught up with the goals they have set themselves in life that they forget how precious life itself is. And some found that the unexpected loss of their health or indeed the loss of a loved one can suddenly turn their lives upside down.

So we can all learn a great lesson from this story: We must all remember next time when we are dwelling on a decision to ask ourselves:

HOW LONG WILL I BE DEAD?

You see this life is so temporary, and so fragile that one can not predict what will happen in the next minute. I did not say next day, or next week, or next year, I just said the next minute and I mean the next minute.

Now let me tell you another story. Please, by the way, have patience and enjoy these stories. They are life-lessons and if you apply what you are going to learn from this book in your daily life, I promise you that you will have much less stress and a much more fulfilling life. You see, stories are very powerful and have a greater effect on our life compared to any other form of learning.

Why? Because in a story you can chose to be the **HERO** or the **VICTIM**. That is absolutely up to you. It is your choice as well as your attitude. It is not down to your education or your upbringing or your cultural background or your family's financial or social status. It all depends on your **ATTITUDE**. Nothing else can make a difference in your life, except your **ATTITUDE** to it.

Excuse Me! Is This Your Body?

You may wish to ask me: 'How do you know this?'

I know this because of my experience with many people over many years – and also by my own experience of having a good attitude. If you like you can now do a little test… Imagine you are reading these pages and not laughing. Well, if you are, that's a little sad. Not because my writing is necessarily very funny, but because you are taking life too seriously and are not enjoying it enough. You need to fix your attitude. Unfortunately there is no mechanic who mends damaged attitudes. The only way you can fix your attitude is to change your negative one for a positive one.

You can't buy a new **POSITIVE MENTAL ATTITUDE** in any shop I know. The only way for you to have a **PMA** is to create it with your own mind, so having said that, let's go back to the story. Did you really think I would forget about the story? No, perhaps not!

Well, this is a story which I heard from a Persian scholar at a Persian conference. Often I think it is a blessing to know more than one language as it gives access to other cultures and people. My wish is that one day there will be one world language and all schools of the world will teach it to the children, and of course our own mother language too. Imagine how smaller the world would become then and how easy communication would be. Sorry, I went off the point again, so let's go back to the story.

And to begin this story you must imagine yourself walking in an endless and empty desert. Are you doing that? Good! Well, while you are walking along, suddenly and unexpectedly you fall into a deep dark hole. And as you are falling down this long dark hole you try to grab something in order to save yourself from falling further.

Eventually you manage to grab something. And after a few moments of desperation and feeling very frightened you begin to see where you are, although it is still very, very dark and it isn't possible for you to see much at all.

As your eyes adjust gradually to the darkness, you find you can now make out the bottom of the hole – and you see that there is a huge dragon down there with its massive mouth wide open ready to swallow anything and everything that may fall down the hole. Then you see that you are holding onto two tree branches, one with each hand, and that your feet are balancing on something, too.

However, when you look closely, you see there is a black mouse chewing the root of the branch on your right-hand side – and a white mouse chewing the root of the branch on your left-hand side. Then you also see that your right foot is resting on a sleeping snake, and your left foot too is standing on another snake.

And still the dragon is waiting for you to arrive below to be swallowed.

As frightening and unbelievable as the story may at first appear, it is in truth not far away from our daily lives. So let me try to analyse the picture for you. The desert is the realm of infinite possibility… The hole is the 'birth canal'… The white and black mice are day and night… And the snakes are chronic or acute diseases or accidents which are waiting to wake up at any moment in our life… Far away below, the gaping-mouthed dragon is the angel of death waiting for the right time. So you tell me: Is our life any different from that picture? I don't really pretend to know the answer to that question. **I simply leave it with you.**

The way I see health is that it is simple and free, and is not appreciated for its right value, on the other hand **DIS-EASE** with all its complexities has become a large business in so many diverse ways that it is almost impossible to see where it is going to end. Focus on dis-ease and ill health only brings more of the same.

The responsibility of people in the health industry must be to educate people to wellness and to take the focus off illness.

My observation has been that when people come to see me I educate them about health and wellness. As a result they begin to understand how important it is for them to take responsibility for their own wellbeing. Now of course when one is unwell they need the support and advice of their physician to regain wellness, but then they also need to be educated on how to stay well.

My vision is that we can change the illness industry into a wellness industry and have very healthy societies who are proactive for their health and not reactive to their illness.

Let's optimistically imagine a picture in our society (since imagination is free why not), which has no ill person. Can you see what is going to happen? One would wonder where all those consultants of all kinds are going to go, and the operating theatres for heart, gallstone, kidney transplants, etc, etc, etc. Also all the companies who make all kinds of instruments for people with various disabilities, and all those insurance companies which are growing like mushrooms everywhere. Wahoo…the list can go on for ever.

Think about what happened when mankind discovered electricity? All it did was developed the society faster but yet at the time people were very nervous of the thought that there would be a loss of jobs because no one would need to buy candles or oil lights.

Did you know that in ancient Persia, the physicians used to get paid by kings and other royals as long as their health was in good shape? As soon as they became ill, the physicians' payments were stopped. Not only their income was under threat, sometimes even their lives were in danger if they were unable to restore the sick to health.

I know that sounds a bit dramatic, but when we look at the societies which have people who live over a hundred years they are more or less operating on the above principles, whereas in most developed countries we are illness victims of a modern mechanical medical system.

Nevertheless, there is one fact which most people agree with and that is complaining, criticising, or condemning, will not bring any good conclusions. Instead a productive and workable suggestion may get us to desirable destinations, that is why I am writing this book and I am hoping this book enables me to reach out to thousands of people, then maybe together we can bring about a wellness programme in the best possible form.

We are
HUMAN BEINGS
Not
HUMAN DOINGS

CHAPTER FOUR

WHERE DOES IT ALL BEGIN?

Once upon a time your Mammy and Daddy started kissing each other and that was the preparation for the start of the world's biggest swimming race. Soon millions of tiny biological sparks that are potential human beings started to swim as fast as they could. Apparently over 350 million individual potential sperm are released in one episode of lovemaking.

And the prize was an egg; what you and 349,999,999 other little biological sparks were swimming for, was this egg. You won and became the little Olympic Gold Medallist out in front of all those other millions of swimmers. From that moment on you became a natural born winner!

Please refer to diagram Number 1 on page 23.

SO YOU ARE, AND CAN GO ON BEING A WINNER IF YOU CHOOSE.

Then you went through the process of the development in your mother's womb for around nine months. At the end of that you took the longest journey that any human can take in this material life – and that is the journey through the birth canal. According to quantum physics it is the longest journey that we ever go through.

Now you are out. And no matter what you are going to do or become, one thing is certain: it is impossible for you to go back to the womb.

And as you start life you are confronted by two things.

- FOOD
- MEDICINE

And the simplest and most important thing I can say to you at this stage of the book is:

LET FOOD BE YOUR MEDICINE AND MEDICINE BE YOUR FOOD.

Where Does It All Begin?

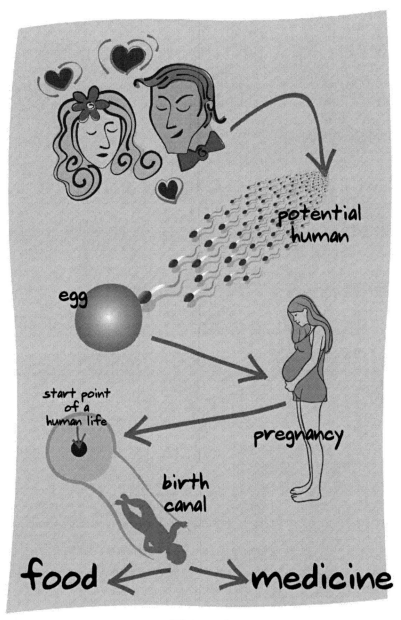

Diagram 1

Excuse Me! Is This Your Body?

Let's start first with **FOOD.** And to do this I ask you please to refer to diagram Number 2 on page 25.

From that you can understand that our body consists of billions of tiny little things called cells. They gather together to make tissue and tissue gathers together to make organs and the combination of organs makes up our body. This is the simplest way we can describe the secret of creation. So for our body to survive, our cells need to be nourished daily with food and water.

As you can see in diagram Number 2 the cycle is as follows:

When cells need energy they send a signal to the brain, in order to act and feed the body.

Through a variety of actions we choose food and enter it to our body.

The food passes through our digestion tract, the nutrition within the food goes to satisfy the cells, and give them the raw material i.e. vitamins minerals protein, etc.

After the cells have been satisfied they send a signal to the brain, the brain then sends a signal to the mouth to stop eating.

This is how we feel full, and stop eating, (Well, we should stop eating; unfortunately we do not always follow this simple law).

This is the survival process of all creatures on the planet.

In fact every creature obeys this law except us.

Maybe that is why human beings are the only species on planet earth that have false teeth.

No other creature, for example, cats, dogs, lions, etc. etc., have false teeth, only human beings. Our dentists suggest to prevent receding gums or tooth decay to do two minutes of brushing and then to floss.

Yet I have never seen cats, dogs, lions or giraffes that do this.

One might say this is because animals eat what they are supposed to, so we must ask ourselves this question, do we eat what we are supposed to eat?

Where Does It All Begin?

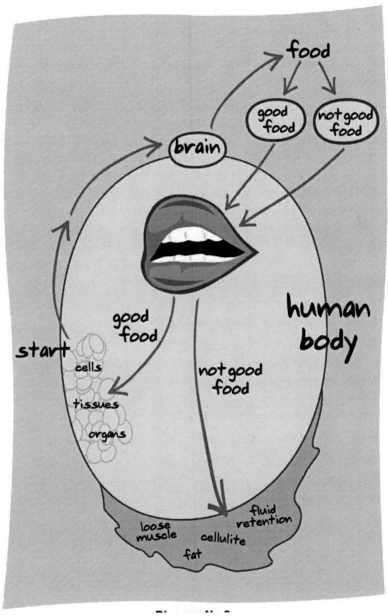

Diagram 2

Let's see where we got lost on the road to well being.

You see, when we consume the right food in the right proportions, everything works according to plan, [the plan being, eating to stay fit and healthy], but usually we do not consume the right foods in the right proportions.

Because there are so many schools of thought about what is right food and what is not, in fact there is not a single food which can be suggested that is right or wrong food. I love that statement (It is not what goes into the mouth that is harmful, but what is coming out). Anyhow this is a vast area that I do not wish to enter into at this moment, but for the purpose of clarification I would like to say that, all the edible substances grown or given to us by Mother Nature in their original state we consider food, for example, apple, seaweed, parsley, etc, etc, are foods in their original state. Other foods not natural, such as aspirin, artificial soft drinks, crisps, and so on, are made by manufacturers, so they need to be put in a different category to original food.

Firstly let me tell you a story, about what is food for one person could be poison for another. The story is called:

TAILORS' MEDICINE IS HARMFUL TO BARBERS.

Once upon a time there was a tailor who was extremely ill; he went to a physician to be cured. The physician examined the man, but could not find out what was wrong with the poor tailor. So he said; I am sorry I do not know what to do with your problem.

The tailor hopelessly asked: Please; give me anything that can bring some comfort.

The physician replied: I am afraid I do not know how to cure your illness.

The man said: If that is the case, I will be dead soon. And he asked the physician: Can I eat something I have always had a desire for but never had the courage to eat it?

The physician asked: What is it that you have a desire to eat.

The tailor replied: I always wanted to eat two kilos of cooked broad beans (also known as fava beans) with a litre of cider vinegar.

The physician paused, for a moment, and then he said: I do not have an objection to this nor can I guarantee that you will be okay.

All night the physician was waiting to hear that the tailor had died.

But to his surprise the man became well. So he wrote in his dairy, the following:

> *Today a tailor came to my clinic; he had an incurable disease, which has been cured by two kilos of cooked broad beans and one litre of cider vinegar.*

A few months later, a barber came to the physician with a problem.

The physician could not find any cure for the barber's problem.

So he told him the story of the tailor with the beans and cider vinegar.

The barber replied: If you think that's what I should do, then I will do it.

So the barber did as the tailor had done and ate two kilos of broad beans and drank one litre of cider vinegar.

After eating, the barber's condition worsened and soon after he died.

On hearing this, the physician wrote in his diary.

> *Yesterday a barber came to my clinic and I had no suggestion for his problem.*
>
> *Because it was a similar problem to a tailor I had seen and he had been cured I suggested that he do the same as the tailor, so he ate two kilos of cooked beans and drank one litre of cider vinegar, and he died. My conclusion as to what we can learn from this is, that foods which can cure tailors are harmful to barbers.*

As silly as the story appears to be there is much wisdom in it.

The point we can learn from this story is that not all foods are suitable for everybody in the same proportions, or, everybody needs different foods or medicine in different proportions. In fact every time I read statistics on health issues I am reminded of that story.

For example, often I have been asked by my clients; is it true that wine is good for us?

Well let us see, is it really? Here is the fact.

Some of the research for studying the effectiveness of wine is being funded by wine companies. Also the main credit has been given to the skin of grapes which has powerful antioxidants that are beneficial chemicals. These are called **Resveratrol** (rĕz-vîr'ĭ-trôl'), a natural compound found in grapes, mulberries, peanuts, plants and other food products, including red wine, that may protect against cancer and cardiovascular disease by acting as an antioxidant, antimutagen, and anti-inflammatory. They also contain phytofactors. Phytonutrient or phytochemicals are all the same things, which are the beneficial components of the fruits and vegetables. Apparently there are over 600 beneficial chemicals or antioxidants in fruits and vegetables and scientists know about only some of them. The latest theory has it, that in fact the colour in fruits and vegetables are the effective part of them. One example is that carrots, oranges, and red peppers, contain large amounts of vitamin C. But the types of vitamin C in each one of them are different and have different effects on us. After all that, the researcher's suggestion is two glasses of 150ml of wine not more than twice a week. In fact more than that has an opposite effect, and also people who are alcoholics should not go near wine! They should consider their condition the same as people who have an allergic reaction to penicillin who tell their doctors about their condition.

Now, my question is this, what is wrong with eating fresh grapes?

I feel we gain more benefits by just eating grapes.

Another example, I have found that people who have problems with acne benefit by drinking the juice of half a lemon in a glass of boiling water with a tea spoon of honey for six weeks, one in the morning and one in the evening before food.

However, this works very well for people who are warm blooded, yet does not have the same effect on cold blooded types.

If you are a teenager and have cold hands and/or cold feet, particularly clammy hands and feet, you would be considered cold blooded, but if you perspire easily especially from shyness and embarrassment you are warm blooded. Please note these are my own observations from many years of experience, I do not have any scientific reference, I would hope to have more information on this in my next book.

Also the environment is another factor that we need to consider for our eating habits.

For example: lemons, oranges, and other yellow fruits are very effective for good health if we live in Spain or Italy, or any Mediterranean countries.

Yet they can have the reverse effect on people who live in Sweden, Denmark, Finland or other Scandinavian countries. Even in England and Ireland, lots of people have allergies to oranges or other citrus fruits. Also many find these types of fruits aggravate their joint pain.

Well, let's go back to the eating. (I bet you thought I'd totally forgotten about what I was talking about! Well, do not worry, this is the Persian style of writing. In fact Mawlana, in the West known as **RUMI**, would jump from one subject to another and then he would be back to it a hundred pages later.)

Why don't we stop eating when we are supposed to?

You see, when we consume food in its original state, our body has control of the amount it needs, and the problem starts from the consumption of processed foods.

Let me give you an example.

If I give you a piece of fruit, or a bowl of porridge, after an adequate amount has been consumed you feel full, and stop eating.

The reason you stop eating is, because your cells are satisfied, and send a signal to the brain which gives an order to the body to stop eating. If you don't stop you will feel nauseous and possibly vomit from over eating.

But this law does not apply when we eat processed food.

Here is an example: When do you know you have eaten enough chocolate, crisps, cake or biscuits, etc, etc?

We don't, and why not? Well, this is a good question.

Here is the reason. If you follow and understand these next few lines, you possibly would never have to diet for the rest of your life.

Processed foods are chemically altered in order to make you consume more of them. Therefore we do not know when to stop eating, for two reasons.

1. There is added fat, sugar or salt, in order to make them tasty, so these added ingredients, confuse the brain as to know when to stop, since they are not satisfactory for the cells nourishment.

2. Most processed foods have artificial ingredients or chemically altered ingredients added to them. This confuses our brain and does not give the message needed to stop eating.

Therefore the cells are still hungry yet we consumed a lot of food. We then store this food in a form of **PARTITIONING FAT** which is usually around the upper arms, abdomen, thighs and hips. That is why we have loose muscle, fat, fluid retention.

Also when we put on weight of two or three stones our organs, like the kidneys, lungs, liver, heart, and so on, are the same weight, and do not increase in size.

So where does the extra weight go?

We keep it in the form of **PARTITIONING FAT** as mentioned before.

(Partitioning fats are the body's way of storing the food surplus so it can be used later, but unfortunately we eat more food before we need to. Homo sapiens like other animals have a specific biological metabolism. Over millions of years of evolution we evolved to our present stage, but nevertheless, the original surviving mechanism remained unchanged. Therefore today like millions of years ago we are responding in the same way, meaning that our body stores some of the food which we consume daily in a form of fat. In simple language because our body does not know when we are going to eat again therefore it stores fat in order to prevent starvation).

That is why one can say:

IN THE WESTERN WORLD PEOPLE ARE OVER FED AND UNDER NOURISHED.

In other words we consume more then we need, also we consume foods which are easily convertible to fat, like lots of processed foods, carbohydrate foods, and sugar.

Now what do you think we do about our over eating and overweight?

Do we start to eat less? Or eat more sensibly? I am afraid the answer is generally no we don't.

We go and buy drugs or supplements which can help us to lose weight and go on a merry-go-round of eating foods which do not feed our cells, and purchase more products to help us lose weight.

So we make our body a dustbin for rubbish we call food and we spend and give away two major valuable assets in our life : our **WEALTH** and our **HEALTH**.

Actually to me **HEALTH** is the most valuable asset we have. Just imagine how much money would you give to get back your health after you have lost it? Of course any amount. Isn't that true? Sure it is. Sorry I got lost and ran away a bit with my horse of passion into the desert of my imagination.

You know I have such a passion to talk about food, medicine and health that I am challenged controlling myself.

So let us get back to the point about what kind of foods we need to look out for or if possible avoid altogether.

I use a letter for some of the foods which are not satisfactory for our body to consume; or at least if you do consume them, do so in minute proportions, I hope this will be helpful for you to easily remember,

The letter is C, a big C. Like chocolate, cake, cream, cookie, champagne, chips, crisps, and the list is endless.

All of the above items, no matter how good their quality or their ingredients, they are types of foods that confuse the metabolic rate of our body.

Please remember, next time when you are eating any of the above food, notice how you are feeling afterward.

Are your cells happy? Or are they crying for:

PROPER FOODS PLEASE!!!!

**Walking
is
Man's
Best Medicine**

Hippocrates

CHAPTER FIVE

THE PROCESS OF DIGESTION

There are two activities that take place during the digestive process which change foods to simple substances and raw materials for use in our body as **ENERGY** and help balance the **HEAT** in the body. These two activities are mechanical action and chemical action.

MECHANICAL ACTION
Chewing and Peristaltic actions are mechanical actions that are responsible for breaking down food into small pieces

CHEMICAL ACTION
This is in two parts. Firstly, as soon as food touches our tongue, a secretion of chemicals such as enzymes, hydrochloric acid and digestive juices are secreted by the pancreas and gallbladder. These enter into the stomach as soon as food goes into our mouth. Sometimes just seeing the food is enough to trigger the above activity. This is called psychological secretion. In fact this is an involuntary response in humans and animals. In early 1900 a Russian scientist called Ivan Petrovich Pavlov did an experiment with dogs. Before feeding the dogs he arranged that a bell would always be rung. After a while each time the bell was rung, the dogs' stomachs secreted digestive juices and they started salivating even when there was no food. Their bodies were responding to a learnt subliminal message.

Having understood this fact, the modern food industry is making millions each year by using this knowledge to encourage us to use processed products, actually going so far as to cause us to become artificially hungry by sending suitable subliminal messages in different ways through advertising in order to encourage us to consume more processed foods.

I hope I am not confusing you, and you are still following me. Here are some examples of these subliminal messages.

The Process of Digestion

Often the TV advertisements for chocolate occur during the break in a movie as a potential aid to relieve the boredom of the break. Or a manufacturer may advertise a breakfast cereal in the late evening. At such times a cool and light nutritional food would be most welcome. But are chocolate and cereals appropriately nutritional at that time for our body?

Here is another example: TV ads often show someone (who looks very healthy!!!) eating sweets or a chocolate bar after finishing work. This consumption of artificial sugars at such a time is a most disturbing action for our digestive tract since this is the very time that our bodies need to have proper nutritional foods rather than processed sugar or any other artificial energy boost that can be absorbed very quickly into our blood stream.

THE BEST CHOICE AT THAT TIME IS A PIECE OF FRUIT OR A BUNCH OF GRAPES

The purpose of the mechanical and chemical digestive actions is to convert foods to recognisable substances for our body to work with. Food will enter our body through the digestive tract via the blood stream from the wall of the stomach, then from the small intestine and lastly from the large intestine. The large intestine is the place where the last part of the nourishment from water and foods will be absorbed, and the rest will pass through the rectum, the anus and out in the form of pulp or faecal matter.

Do you know that large amounts of the foods that we eat actually pass right through us? And only very small amounts of foods are absorbed! And even that amount is exchanged and replaced with dead cells within 60 to 120 days? So isn't it sensible to reduce the amount we consume and try to overcome the artificial hunger which we are being programmed with everyday?

Let me now give you a little demonstration of psychological chemical secretion. Just visualise yourself in the kitchen. You are cutting a fresh, juicy lemon and you are going to squeeze the juice into your mouth. If you do this action just by your imagination, you will experience a secretion of saliva in your mouth which is ready to help the lemon juice to be digested in your stomach. Now if I ask you to visualise that you are eating a piece of pounded yam most of you will have no saliva in your mouth at all – unless you are an African who knows about the smell and flavour of pounded yam and your salivary glands are thus stimulated by that memory.

People often say to me: 'But Abbas, I love chocolate, or I love cheese cake, or I love cappuccino or…'

'No my dear', I must say to you, 'Sadly, you are being trained to love these substances. I do not love those things, because in my time and in my country we were not taught to love them. Instead we were taught to love other things.'

* * * * * * * *

Now I would like to give you some suggestions for improving your eating habits. You may consider these twelve suggestions as a collection of guidelines.

- Before eating pause for a few moments and thank the creator.
- No matter how small , always try to eat some breakfast
- Don't eat unless you are hungry.
- Make sure you chew your foods well before swallowing.
- Try to avoid foods that are hard to chew.
- Start with liquid food, then soft food, then heavy food.
- After eating, take a short walk so the food can settle in your stomach.
- Never do heavy exercise on a full stomach.
- Don't eat unless your last meal has been digested.
- Do not consume two foods that go against each other.
- Fasting some time during the year is great for our wellbeing.
- Don't read or look at television while you are eating.

The above guidelines come from Persian and Arabic writings. They are suitable for anybody on any diet, in any country or culture. I feel I was blessed to come across these writings in my life. I wish I could say I am applying those 100% myself, but I must confess that I am not. However I am working towards that goal every day.

I have noticed during my years of practice helping to improve people's health that they either eat badly from habit or a lack of knowledge about food. Whichever it is, ill health can be adjusted by educating yourself or by changing bad eating habits. Good eating habits can be easily learned and we can then apply them in our daily lives to stay healthy. It is like learning our own phone numbers. After repeating them a few times, we know them by heart

Now I will give you a short explanation of each of the above twelve guidelines. Much as I would love to provide an in-depth explanation of each one, I know that this book would then become thousands of pages. So here goes:

Ideally you only need to know them as I mentioned above, but for some of you who wish to know why those guide lines are important, I will now give some additional explanation about them.

GUIDELINE 1
Before eating pause for a few moments and thank the creator.
This is one of the most important guidelines that I feel we should know about eating. The application of this guideline separates humans from any other animal. The implications of this principle will bring blessings to our body, mind and soul. This helps us to become aware of our surroundings and helps us to realise how much effort it may have taken to prepare the food that is in front of us. So start in the name of creation and finish by expressing gratitude that the food is available for us.

GUIDELINE 2
No matter how small, always try to eat some breakfast
Eating a small amount of breakfast with wholegrain foods or some pieces of fruit is much healthier then eating a large breakfast or a breakfast of rich foods. When we eat a large breakfast, huge amounts of our blood supply goes to the digestive tract in order to digest the food. This reduces the blood supply left for our other organs. There is also the

possibility that rich foods in the morning or a large amount of food for breakfast can cause us to tire easily.

On the other hand if we do not consume any breakfast at all our bodies do not have enough calories to support the day's activities. SO A BREAKFAST CONSISTING OF A SMALL AMOUNT OF WHOLE GRAIN FOODS OR FRUITS IS HIGHLY RECOMMENDED.

GUIDELINE 3
Do not eat unless you are hungry

This is the simplest of all these guidelines. Yet we often fail to apply it in our lives. In fact through the power of advertising and our experience of constantly being bombarded by posters, TV commercials, and other forms of food advertising, our taste buds are constantly being encouraged to ask for foods that we really do not need to consume at such times.

Here briefly I would like to tell you that the first health paper that I wrote about food started like this: **The joy of foods are only experiences in our mind.**

The article was only a few pages long and I would like to share a small part of it with you now, as I feel the key points are very relevant to this guide.

Imagine a time when you were very, very hungry, and the food in front of you appeared delicious. And now imagine that you have eaten the delicious food and you are full. Think carefully!! If the same food was placed in front of you again immediately, do you think you would still see it as being delicious in the same way? Of course not! You would not have any desire for it at all!

I remember very vividly the time when I was writing that article. It was after I had done a special four-day fast which allows you to have as much as you like of one kind of fruit or vegetable juice and plenty of water. In fact, that was the recommendation of the Holistic Healing and Herbal Medicine School at which I was studying at the time. The school recommended that we should fast and continue with our usual daily activities and then write down our views about foods and the effects different foods have on us. On the last day of my fast I was walking in town. As I passed a fast food take away van, the smell was absolutely irresistible. So I decided that when I finished my swimming, I would go home and prepare a vegetarian burger.

It was interesting to notice that during the whole forty minutes of my swimming exercise, I was thinking of the burger I was going to have and how juicy and tasty it was going to be! When I arrived home and cooked my burger it was tasty and juicy just as I thought it would be. Contrary to that, if I would have eaten a burger every day the chance of enjoying it in the same way would be very unlikely. From that experience I now know why a common saying exists around the world that: **Hunger is the best appetiser**

This thought about hunger leads me naturally into another story called *A HUNGRY MAN ARRIVES IN A VILLAGE* and it goes like this:.

One day a strange man with poor clothing arrived in a village. He was so hungry that he ran straight to the village bakery. There he asked for some bread to eat since he had walked a long way without any food. The baker asked for payment first but the poor man raised his hands in supplication.

'Please, please,' he begged, 'I am so hungry and I don't have any money. You have to give me some bread.'

The baker thought for a moment before replying. Then he said: 'OK, I will make a deal with you. If you can give me something else other than money – it can be anything – I will accept it and give you some bread.'

The stranger replied: 'I have nothing, nothing at all...except, I suppose, my faith.'

The baker looked at him again thoughtfully. 'OK,' he said at last. 'If you will sell me your faith, I will give you some bread.'

The poor man looked startled. Then realising he had no other choice he made a deal to sell his faith for a loaf of fresh bread. He received the bread gratefully and sat down, there and then and ate it as fast as he could. He enjoyed every last bit of it then stood up and said: 'Thanks be to God! My faith is back to me again.'

The baker shook his head, 'No,' he argued. 'You sold your faith to me for a loaf of bread. Have you forgotten already?'

The poor man looked at the baker and smiled suddenly. *'Well my friend, surely you should know that, the hungry man does not have any faith.'*

I hope you can appreciate the moral of this story. In Persian culture this tale is very meaningful, and is often used in political circumstances. However please don't let yourself be so hungry that you will do anything for a loaf of bread.

GUIDELINE 4
Make sure you chew your foods well before swallowing.

This is one of the most important eating habits that we must apply in order to have a healthy digestive tract. These days people suffer from so many digestion problems and most can be avoided by applying this simple guideline. I have seen so many people who followed this simple principle and gained great relief from indigestion and digestive disorders such as **I.B.S** (Irritable Bowel Syndrome), heartburn, hiatus hernia and others.

So, simply chew your foods very well – and swallow it only when it's almost a liquid.

GUIDELINE 5
Try to avoid foods that are hard to chew..

This guideline is good for the wellbeing of our teeth and our digestive tracts. So avoid chewing hard sweets, dry nuts, and uncooked meat or any other food which is hard to chew. Eating dry hard nuts is not advisable, since they are also hard for the digestive tract to break down. You can either eat them after soaking them overnight, in pure clean water, at room temperature or take them cooked in food, for example you can cook the nuts with rice and they will be very tasty, especially cashew nuts.

GUIDELINE 6
Start with liquid food, then soft food, then heavy food.

Start your meal with water or juices if they are cold. Then go on to soups or fruits like melons. Then take cooked foods i.e. protein source or carbohydrate foods. Finally move to the desserts or cakes.

The Process of Digestion

Here I would like to sound a note of warning: **NEVER, NEVER, NEVER, NEVER** eat a burger or chips or any other heavy foods on their own if you wish to have a healthy digestive tract. It is absolutely vital that you have some liquid first, especially when you are hungry and have an empty stomach.

This is in fact a quite complex guideline to understand, so I will do my best to simplify it. When our stomach is empty or between our regular meal times, our inner stomach actually shrinks and stays in a form of layer's like an accordion or like curtains. So when we drink some water, particularly if we do so half an hour before taking food, our body sends the water back to our stomach from our inner reserved water, and this gives us several beneficial digestive aids. For further details about this, please refer to the section on water that gives a fuller explanation or you can refer to Dr.B's book *Your Body's Many Cries for Water*.

Also when we eat food without drinking water first, we require much more food before we feel full. Sometimes it takes the stomach fifteen minutes or more to start digesting the food. That is why we may experience pain in our stomach when we eat food fast or eat dry and heavy foods.

As well as this we need to know that there is a valve or sphincter at the end part of the stomach called the **PYLORUS**, which is a tube-shaped part of the stomach that angles from the main part of the stomach toward the first segment of the small intestine. During eating time the **PYLORUS** needs to stay closed and it is also very sensitive to liquid, especially cold liquid. That is why we need to learn the habit of drinking liquid before our foods, not during or after meals, unless it is about a half or one hour after eating. Otherwise the undigested food will pass through and bring about other digestive complications.

So to repeat the essentials of this guideline, when we eat, it is important to follow the sequence of having **liquid first, soft foods second and heavy foods last** if we wish to have a healthy digestive tract.

GUIDELINE 7
After eating, take a short walk so the food can settle in your stomach.
I do not think we need to say much about this, since this is common

sense. But nonetheless I need to make sure you know why this is important. We need to use the above combinations of knowledge with the following in mind: walking can bring about the settlement of foods in the stomach especially when we walk in a temperature cooler than the eating area. In fact, Hippocrates, who is widely regarded as the father of modern medicine said very wisely: **Walking is man's best medicine.**

GUIDELINE 8
Never do heavy exercise on a full stomach.
Again this is a very clear and simple guideline. I mention it only to bring its importance to your attention so that I can be sure that you are aware of this.

GUIDELINE 9
Don't eat unless your last meal has been digested.
You might ask yourself how I can follow this guideline No 9 and guideline No 3 (which directs us not to eat unless we are hungry). Well here is an example:

Imagine a day when you have finished your main meal. About an hour has passed and you feel hungry again. This could be for several reasons. One reason may be that you have been exposed to some appetising looking food again – or you have been trapped again in the net of food advertising. You see technically speaking you should not be hungry and so you may be artificially hungry or possibly you haven't really learned the difference between hunger and thirst. So in order to know the difference just drink a glass or two of, pure clean, water then wait for a few minutes to see how you feel.

GUIDELINE 10
Do not consume two foods that war against each other.
This is actually a very interesting guideline and from what I have observed since I left Persia, this dietary principle is not well understood in the West. Why do I say this? Well, I will begin by asking you to think of what is one of the most common fast food shops in the Western world, or perhaps I should say, the Developed World? That's right– Fish and Chips. Actually I had better not go into too much detail on this subject as it would take another whole book to explain this issue alone. But in simple terms it is important that we know our stomach's pH level.

The Process of Digestion

What is pH? Technically speaking, pH stands for the Power of Hydrogen. Broken down into the simplest form, our bodies are composed of carbon, oxygen and hydrogen. The pH is a measurement of the action of hydrogen and the balance of acidity and alkalinity in the living system. Our bodies are a living system. When testing pH, the resulting measurement used is a number anywhere from 0 to 14. The neutral level is 7, with lower numbers representing an acidic state of balance, and higher representing an alkaline state. It is best for our stomachs to operate at levels between 7 and 8. This means that the stomach should be primarily alkaline with mild acidity.

When we eat protein foods like fish, our stomach produces acid to break it down. Then the next mouthful might be a carbohydrate food like chips or potatoes and the stomach has to change immediately to an alkaline environment in order to convert the carbohydrate to sugar for absorption into our blood stream. Again we eat another piece of fish or meat that is protein and the stomach's PH needs to switch quickly back again to acid to break it down and this goes on until we finish our meal. Our stomach is in grave stress after we have eaten in this way because the stomach PH level is going up and down like a yo-yo. We should always eat in a way which prevents the stomach from being forced into rapid change of PH activity.

There is a great possibility that people, who consume foods which stimulate this sort of oscillation, are eating foods that are not in harmony with each other and this can often cause them to feel tired very easily. Please note that many vegetarian dishes do not have this problem because proteins from beans, pulses, nuts, seeds, grains and similar things do not require acidity in the stomach to break them down.

Well I think you may see now that this is one of the worst habits that many people have acquired – and it is not easy to break. There are books written about this subject which is called 'food combining' but the purpose of this brief guideline is to explain the two most common types of food – protein and carbohydrate – which disagree with each other, and that we should avoid eating together. One other example of this could be having a citric drink with dairy products in the same meal or part of a meal. So avoid drinking orange or grapefruit juice with your breakfast cereal which has milk in it. However to keep it very simple, remember the best dish is always: **Single, simple food.**

For now, let's leave it like that and go on to the next important piece of knowledge!

GUIDELINE 11
Fasting some time during the year is great for our wellbeing.
I will mention here just a few reasons why we can benefit from fasting

Have you ever tried to feed dogs or cats when they are sick? What do they do?

They have a rest and a fast. Just look at it this way: we have holidays during the year or we take a day off during the week. So isn't it just as sensible to give a break to our digestive system?

I believe it to be very necessary – but you may say: 'Abbas, if we fast, won't we possibly suffer from malnutrition'?

My reply to that is: 'My dear, believe me, in the Western world we consume more than we should.'

I know I may appear to be making a judgement here but when we look at any of the world religions and their traditions, we see the importance of fasting has always been taught. Fasting can also be offered as a last resort when there is a terminal illness on the agenda. Many people have been cleared from their terminal illness by following fasting principles alone. There are many ways in which one can fast and here I will give you just a few ideas:

- Fast for one day a week. During this day drink two or more litres of water and take nothing else, starting after breakfast until the following morning.
- Fast on one type of juice alone for three, seven, fourteen or twenty-one days – or even twenty-eight days – based on the intensity of the health problems you are faced with.
- Fast the same way as above but with grapes and water alone
- Fast on brown rice, with soy sauce or yoghurt if desired, for three to ten days maximum.

- Fast for a few days during spring or autumn.
- Finally just try to do some form of fasting to clear your body from toxins.

GUIDELINE 12
Don't read or look at television while you are eating.
I wish I could say that I always obey this guideline. But unfortunately I do not apply this principle 100% of the time myself and occasionally watch TV while I am eating. So you can see that I too, need to work on improving this. But I can definitely say that I never read while I am eating.

Why is it beneficial, you may be wondering, to apply this guideline? Well the fact is that when we read or watch TV whilst eating, our mind creates different sensations in our body. Therefore, our mind does not fully appreciate what we are eating and cannot respond to the creation of relevant enzymes which we need to digest the foods we are consuming. Also, while our mind is busy reading or watching TV we pour undigested food down into our colon. That is why lots of people suffer from allergy reactions to foods.

Those then are the essential guidelines to maintaining a healthy and efficient digestive tract. To conclude this chapter I just wish to say: when you have learned how to apply all above guidelines, not only will you have a healthy digestive tract, you will also have much more energy, you will have a good sleeping pattern and you will generally feel much better in every way.

So do try to apply all these essential guidelines as much as possible. You may need to change a few deeply entrenched habits to do so but the benefits will be well worth any effort you make. When we don't apply the above guidelines we create **DIS-EASE** and **ILLNESS** which I am going to talk about next. But overall we need to make up our minds to follow Hippocrates who once famously said:

Let food be your medicine and medicine be your food.

The driving force of
ILLNESS
is
FEAR

The driving force of
HEALTH
is
FAITH

CHAPTER SIX

ILLNESS AND WELLNESS – THE CONNECTIONS

Now that I have discussed food and our eating habits in a brief but comprehensive way, I will discuss medicine and what the connections are between **ILLNESS** and **WELLNESS**. With the help of the Illness-Wellness Chart on this page we will consider how these are interlinked and how we can become the victim of **ILLNESS** by not following proper eating habits and abusing our bodies in other ways.

But first we need to have some form of yardstick to measure the reality of illness so that we can develop our understanding of what illness is and of how and why we get trapped in it. Please refer to Diagram Number 3 on the next page for a better understanding of my meanings.

Illness-Wellness Chart

ILLNESS	WELLNESS
FEAR	FAITH
ANXIETY	HOPE
REACTIVE MEDICINE	PROACTIVE MEDICINE
SADNESS	HAPPINESS
NO RESPONSIBILITY	TAKE RESPONSIBILITY
POWERLESS	POWERFUL
RESTRICTION	FREEDOM
PAIN	JOY

Please feel free dear reader, to add words representing your own individual experiences to either side

Excuse Me! Is This Your Body?

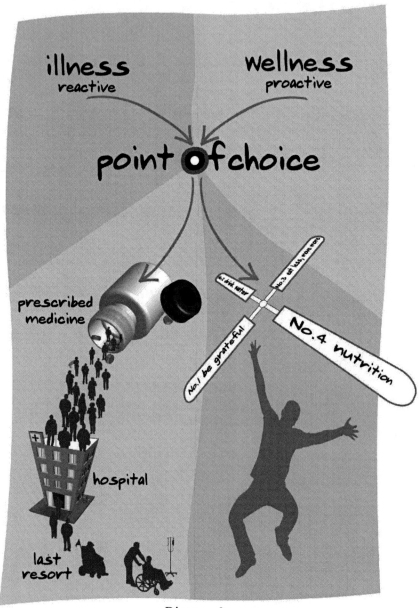

Diagram 3

Illness and Wellness – The Connections

As we can see in the left column of the Chart on page 47, everything there can be described as negative and everything in the right column as positive or rewarding. Let's consider these things one by one.

The left Illness column begins with **FEAR** and the equivalent right-hand Wellness column begins with **FAITH**. **FEAR** grows from anxiety about the seriousness of any **DISEASE** and it is obviously more beneficial if faith in some form can be brought to bear. I love the following quotation from a writer who said in her book:

FAITH IS NOT SOMETHING YOU DISCOVER, IT IS SOMETHING YOU DEVELOP.

The left column continues with **ANXIETY** while on the right under Wellness there is **HOPE**. I am sure that you will agree with me that most women waiting for the results of a smear test or mammogram or blood test will feel anxious while they are waiting. Very few would admit to feeling relaxed during that waiting period.

Then we are reminded that in Illness there is **PAIN**, in Wellness there is **JOY**. Do I need to elaborate on this? I do not think so.

I wish I could examine thoroughly all of the Illness and Wellness issues, but then this book will become a complex text book and you would be using it as a door stop rather than hopefully reading it as a joyful and light teaching story book. However, the most important heading of all is **RESPONSIBILITY**, which goes hand and hand with **POWER**. You see, when we welcome responsibility we gain power. As simple as this may appear to be, most of us fail to embrace this simple principle.

Let me tell you another little story to elaborate my point better. This one might be called:

THE STORY OF SOLOMON, KING AND PROPHET, THE MOSQUITO AND THE WIND

According to the story, Solomon, who was both a King and a Prophet, was able to speak the language of all the living creatures in his land. So one day a mosquito came to Solomon's palace, complaining about the strength of the wind. The mosquito also complained about the injustice of the wind's cruel and inconsiderate behaviour towards poor weak creatures like itself and other insects.

So King Solomon asked the mosquito to sit down beside him and called the wind to his palace. The wind eventually arrived at Solomon's palace with a loud noise and a dance of glory and at that moment the mosquito disappeared.

So King Solomon asked the wind: 'Why are you so cruel and inconsiderate to some creatures who try to live in my kingdom?'

'If it pleases your Majesty,' the wind replied respectfully, 'this is not my fault, it is my nature. I have been created to clear the air of negative energy and bring refreshment into the atmosphere. I am only passing through with my natural flow. I am not trying to destroy anything.'

'Hmm,' mused King Solomon, 'I suppose you have a point there,'

'Yes I certainly do,' the wind continued. , 'Furthermore it is the duty of the mosquito and other small creatures to be strong. Also, let me ask you this: 'How could it be possible for wind and mosquito to sit down side by side on one throne?' The wind paused for effect, and then concluded sonorously. 'Mosquito stays when I am not around. But when I arrive mosquito must go!'

The humour of this story, as simple as it appears, is closely related to our daily life. There is a hidden message in it.

For example, I often have patients who would like to have a healthy body and lots of energy, but they are not prepared to give up their undesirable habits. I vividly remember a lady who came to me complaining of a recurrent and persistent cough.

So I asked her: 'Do you smoke?'

She replied: 'Oh please don't ask me to give up my cigarettes.'

I asked her: 'How many cigarettes do you smoke?'

'Forty a day,' she said quietly.

I asked if she could reduce them. 'No,' she said.

So do you see we can't do anything if we won't accept the consequences of our own actions? So this is what I said to the lady: 'You are actually wasting your time and money by coming to me if you are not prepared

Illness and Welllness – The Connections

to meet me half way in changing habits that are harmful to you and causing your cough.'

Cases like this have led me to conclude that many of us confuse the difference between problems themselves and the cause of the problems. In my humble opinion, I must say that:

It is not heart dis-ease, cancer, high blood pressure or other chronic diseases that are killing people. It is the abuse of cigarettes, alcohol, and poor nutrition, which is the cause of the majority of our complicated chronic diseases that are killing us.

As I go on I will explain further the links between Illness and Wellness and it will become more obvious what I mean when I say: '**WE GAIN POWER**' when we follow the Wellness principle.

To sum up, it can be said that the Goal of Medicine must be focused firmly upon:

STAYING HEALTHY DURING THE WELLBEING PERIOD AND RESTORING HEALTH IN THE TIME OF ILLNESS.

So let's get on with it.

Imagine you are exactly on middle point, between Illness and Wellness on the chart. In other words, you are not ill but you do not feel well either. So you go to your doctor, and seek his or her help. You might start like this:

'Doctor, I do not feel well. My legs hurt and I can't see as well as I used to. Also I get tired easily.'

Your doctor might say: 'Oh, you're ageing, that's all!'

Or perhaps they might think that the combination of your symptoms indicates a particular pathology or patterns of symptoms associated with a particular disease. The doctor will then prescribe a medicine which will take care of the problems.

Please note this is only intended to be a general example and should not be considered as an exact account of a visit to a doctor.

Now I am going to give another example: Just for argument's sake, let's say your doctor might diagnose you with the problem of high blood pressure and prescribe the relevant medicine in order to take care of that problem. Let's say the medicine works and you are happy and the doctor is also happy. Now you have to take that medicine for the rest of your life because as soon as you stop taking the medicine, your problems return.

Funnily enough a high percentage of people have no problem in taking drugs with a powerful and possibly uncomfortable or damaging side effect for the rest of their life, but they argue about taking a nutritional supplement, which in the long run could protect them from Illness.

It would appear that the purpose of most prescribed medicine is not to cure problems but relieve the patient's symptoms. This means there's a good chance that the patients will become dependent on that drug for the rest of their life.

Now that is the good news.

You might say: 'If that is the good news, what is the bad news?

Well the bad news varies between the following two possibilities:

- the prescribed medicine does not relieve the problems
- the prescribed medicine has side-effects

Let us examine these one by one. When in the first case the prescribed medicine does not work, often your doctor will prescribe another one and yet another one until they find a medication that will work. An alternative might be that you get fed up and go to a different doctor – if you can.

In the second case the side effects of the drugs prescribed are the main problem.

Did you know that:

THERE IS HARDLY ANY PRESCRIBED OR NON–PRESCRIBED DRUG ON THE MARKET WHICH DOES NOT HAVE A SIDE EFFECT

Let's say you are given a drug for high blood pressure and the side effect is that you get migraine headache. You then go to your doctor who will,

Illness and Wellness – The Connections

more than likely, prescribe a drug for your migraine headache. As funny as it seems, hardly any doctor will say that the drug first given to you caused the migraine headache.

So you go home with two drugs one for blood pressure and one for migraine headache. A few days, weeks or months later, or maybe a few years later, you have other side effects from the drugs, like constipation, and your doctor will give you something for your constipation, and the story goes on until you are totally fed up and still do not feel well.

How could you feel well with all those drugs inside you anyway? If you have never experienced this kind of scenario you will perhaps think I am writing a comic story. But sadly it is all true

Yet even now all that is still the good news!

And again you may say: 'If this is the good news, what is the bad news?'

Well the bad news is that your problem still remains the same and a few more problems have been added to the original problem.

So this is now the time that you visit the doctor again and he or she seeks yet another solution to your problems. You are sent to a specialist or somewhere else for more tests – or even worse you end up in hospital. My experience has been very similar in most of the countries in which I have lived and travelled, including Iran, Pakistan, Israel, Africa, Russia, Uzbekistan, Holland, Germany, England, Northern Ireland and the Irish Republic. Almost all of these countries have hospitals full or near to full capacity. My experiences tell me that in most countries of the world; more or less the same story exists. I have a feeling that you will agree with me in making this statement. If not, I would love to hear from you, on how your country deals with this issue.

Now if you ask people who are hospitalised for whatever reason, they will tell you they do not want to be there. Nobody wants to be in that situation. Yet we only have to look around, read, see, or to experience for ourselves the long queues, the long waiting lists for hospitals that are overflowing.

We also have to take heed of the fact that the Health Budgets of most countries are being swallowed up by the cost of drugs that are being prescribed. So, all of the health budgets of our countries are under severe pressure. Please remember that this is not because of negligence or carelessness on the part of the medical doctors or nurses. I personally have some close friends and associates who are either medical doctors or nurses and all of them are working at full capacity and with full-hearted good intentions.

At the end of the day they are all people, just like you and me. Yet the amount of pressure on the people who are in the medical care profession is unbelievably great. Most of them are totally exhausted by the overwork that has been imposed on them. I would like to say from the bottom of my heart that I have the highest respect for their integrity and hard work, for which many of them receive very little recognition or reward.

So clearly we need to look at other options and alternative choices that can be made, instead of the never-ending and constant prescribing of drugs. One definition of insanity I like which is very telling:

DOING THE SAME THING REPEATEDLY AND EXPECTING A DIFFERENT RESULT EACH TIME.

So isn't it time for change?

Well in my opinion change is well overdue. We need to look urgently at other ways of taking care of public health alongside the current medical system. **I have at least a thousand and one workable suggestions for ways that the mainstream system might work alongside alternative therapies.**

First and foremost the most important one is the establishment of **WELLNESS HOMES** which I will be discussing near the end of the book, but for now I will give you some other examples which make my point a bit clearer.

One of the suggestions I can recommend to you is the philosophy and work of Dr. Ray Strand's practice and his writings. He wrote a book called *What Your Doctor Doesn't Know About Nutritional Medicine May Be Killing You*. Dr. Strand himself has been a general medical practitioner for almost 27 years. In his book he describes many known

Illness and Wellness – The Connections

degenerative diseases where, with the combined help of modern medicine and nutrition, the restoration of patients' health becomes apparent. For each disease he describes the cases of real people who have been healed as examples. These types of examples are so many among some of the medical profession, who are trying to change the old way and are open minded and their true interest is the wellbeing of their patients.

Another area where I am hoping for change is within governments and their policies. Well let's hope some Minister for Health somewhere soon rises to his or her feet and says: **'I am going to change this system'**. This would be a good start.

Why?

Because governments are paying the bills, at least they are paying the bills with money out of their Health Budgets, which ultimately comes out of every taxpayer's pocket. But none of them are brave enough to act and do something with the present self-governing and self-policing professional medical systems. Would you believe it if I told you that right now there are thousands of medical doctors who wish that they could be allowed to use other forms of treatment alongside their mainstream, so-called modern medical systems?

Some of the braver ones are working towards changing the health care system. But still large portions of the health care budget, which in reality is the people's wealth and taxpayers' money, could be used much more beneficially focusing on wellness rather than illness.

So I am going to declare here that one of my greatest dreams is that firstly copies of these few pages of this book that you are reading now will somehow find their way into the hands of Health Ministers in as many countries of the world as possible. The second part of that dream is that some or all of them will apply the principles outlined here to their Health Care systems. I know that ultimate dream can come true, because if one or more Health Ministers take even a small first step, the result would be beyond our imaginings.

For example, let's say the Minister of Health in the Republic of Ireland decides to place water filters in just one hospital or a small number of our hospitals and gives instructions to the nurses that every hour some patients would be given two glasses of **PURE, CLEAN, CLEAR,** water, from 8 am to 6 pm. This would be done with the supervision of doctors in the case of particular conditions for certain patients. Then the next step would be to monitor and compare the outcome of those patients who receive this daily water intake and compare results with patients in other hospitals which are not following this routine and see what happens.

My feeling is the result will be a great success and a very high percentage of the patients will feel a considerable benefit. I know from my own experience of treating people that when they drink water in similar amounts their conditions improve more than fifty percent.

So why do we not do this officially? What have we got to lose? In the Republic of Ireland alone the Health Care budget is over 10 billion euro a year. Let us say one million euros of it be spent on this project. That is no more than .0001 per cent of the budget because 100 million euro is only one percent. Moreover, water does not generally interfere with most medications or pathologies as far as I know – although it is important to note that there are a small number of exceptions.

So what I am saying plainly is that there is a way that all of us can help promote health and wellness more widely in our own countries by taking such an important initial action. Yes, we can each of us photocopy these pages and mail them to the Health Minister of our country asking that these suggestions and proposals be considered and put into action. Imagine if ten or twenty thousand letters arrived in your Health Minister's office. What is the possibility that the minister might take some action? I would guess in those circumstances the chances might be as high as ninety-nine percent. .

Some two years ago I read the marvellous and very important 'water cure' book by Dr Fereydoon Batmanghelidj my outstanding fellow countryman. His original book is entitled *Your Body's Many Cries for Water* and I write more about it and 'Dr Batman' or 'Dr B' as he is widely and affectionately known in Chapter Nine of this book and in an Appendix at the end of the book on great healers of the past and present. After reading the book I immediately purchased many copies and sent them to various people who were in high positions and could make decisions about people's health. I did not wait to see what other people were doing, I took action.

I know now his British publisher, The Tagman Press, which is also publishing this new book, had been doing the same thing in the United Kingdom and encouraging its readers to do likewise. So if we all continue to take action, we will surely succeed. If we do nothing, things will not change.

However aiming to convince governments is only one part of this mission. We know as I have said above that the Health Care systems of all countries are greatly influenced by the big pharmaceutical companies who have enormous financial resources and power. So what do we have to do? Should we start fighting with those big pharmaceutical companies? No, that would be a silly thing to do. Besides, it is almost impossible to fight with these giant companies. It would be like ants trying to fight with a dragon. Also fighting is never a good thing to do, no matter how good the cause. In truth, nobody can win with a fighting spirit. We need to act wisely and responsibly. So here are some of my own suggestions. As a first step **we must starve them!**

How can we starve them? Well by freeing ourselves from the unnecessary use of drugs. The question is how can we free ourselves from the unnecessary use of drugs?

First by being healthy ourselves.

Second we need to teach others how to become healthy so the wellness principle can spread faster around the world

And you will no doubt say: 'But Abbas, we need drugs and we need hospitals.'

My reply is. 'Yes, of course we do need some drugs, but not that many. And yes, we do need hospitals – but again different kinds of hospitals.'

- We need a type of hospital to take care of us when we have accidents and emergency.

- We need a type of hospital to teach us how to become healthy – and also how to remain healthy.
- We need a type of hospital that has indoor and outdoor swimming pools.
- We need hospitals that serve wholesome organically grown food in their kitchens.
- We need a type of hospital that gives us correct dosages and information about nutritional supplements.
- We need hospitals with all kinds of gyms – and trainers to teach us how to become fit and healthy.
- We need hospitals with at least two medical people for each patient.

Please note the above few suggestions are parallel to Wellness Home principles

When hospitals begin to operate in such a way and patients become well (relatively drug free) they will be longing for the freedom of life outside the confines of the hospital environment and will have gained the knowledge how to sustain wellbeing as much as possible. You may say this is too much to ask for. But do you know that even with only 10% of the existing expenditures, all the above and much more can be achieved, when we concentrate on **WELLNESS** instead of **ILLNESS?**

That is what the word 'hospital' really means anyway. It is the place where we need to be given hospitality, not a place that is overcrowded and has perpetually overworked staff. Do they make mistakes as a result of their tiredness? Of course they do! They are human beings for heaven's sake! And all humans are prone to making mistakes. I have made so many mistakes while I am typing these lines, but nobody gets harmed by such mistakes. If a poor tired doctor or nurse makes a mistake in hospital, it could cost someone their life. They have huge responsibility and are working under tremendous pressures and for very long hours.

As I said before in Chapter Three:

Did you know that in ancient Persia, the physicians used to get paid by

kings and other royals as long as their health was in good shape? As soon as they became ill, the physician's payments were stopped. Not only their income was under threat, sometimes even their lives were in danger if they were unable to restore the sick to health.

I often wonder what would happen if in the Western world the medical system tried to operate the same way. I think more than half of the doctors would become dependent on social welfare payments.

Anyway here is my point; we all need to be educated about **HEALTH** and **WELLNESS** – that is what we are missing. Then, when we are educated, we need to take action. If you read these pages and sigh, nothing will happen. You need to do something….anything which is **GOOD, RIGHT**, and **TRUE.** When our actions are directed by good intentions, like those mentioned above, we will have a good system in a very short period of time.

We need to support each other and to co-operate with each other in order to survive. You tell me, what is it that is stopping us from doing the same in our **HEALTHCARE** system? All of us need to get involved.

You might say: 'But what can I do?'

Well, you can in reality do a lot. You would not believe how much power is in your hands right now. All you have to do is to recognise it, be aware of it and act on the information received. For example:

Did you know that over 150 pathologies or symptoms of disease in the human body are caused by nothing more than a lack of calcium? For example these conditions include osteoporosis, backache, PMS, arthritis, and Bell's palsy.

Did you know that a high percentage of all **DIS-EASES** are due to nothing more than nutrition deficiency?

Now that you do know, you can take your own independent action to seek remedies. The list of the many illnesses that can be overcome via nutrition and wellness programmes is endless. This brings up the question: Can nutrition cure all diseases?

Well I do not like to use the word cure, for two reasons.

First when we say cure that means it is permanent. No pharmaceutical drug has ever been produced to do that anyway. Remember that the drugs that are prescribed for different ailments only settle the symptoms. They never cure the underlying problems.

Second, if I say I can cure, then a book such as this, would not be in front of you, because nobody would publish it and they would be right not to.

Yet if you look at these lines and think about them objectively you will understand that not only can we be free from these diseases but also these diseases need never exist. Also you can read and study what I have studied through The Lancet medical journal or TheLancet.com and other similar medical researches which are freely available in your local library or on the internet. I think then you would do for your health exactly what I am doing for mine, which is focusing on wellness.

I would like to share with you a story, but first let me say this about acquiring information. Sometimes having it can make us confused, and feel unsure as to what is right or wrong for our health, sometimes one can say, I was better off when I knew nothing. This is not so. This is your body and you deserve to know how to treat it well so that you have a good place to live. After all it is the only body you have, for all of your life.

Just remember the purer the substances you put into your body the better chance you have of good health. So inform yourself of what is being suggested to you, and take responsibility for your actions. You will feel much better about yourself and your health.

Now let me tell you that story:

THE STORY OF A MULLAH AND HIS BEARD.
Once upon a time there was a Mullah living in a city in Iran. The term 'Mullah' is a symbolic venerated person in Old Persian storybooks. Well one day this Mullah was walking gracefully in the street and he arrived at the market to do some shopping. The merchant with whom he was dealing asked him this question.

'Dear Mullah, I am wondering if you can help me with something that I am curious about?'

Illness and Welllness – The Connections

The Mullah replied, 'Sure, I will if I can. What is it?'

He said: 'You see, my friend, and myself were talking about your beard, and how nice a beard it is. We know that it must take you so much time to take care of it, but there was one thing that puzzled us and we could not come to an agreement about it. At night when you go to sleep, do you put your beard above your blanket or under your blanket?'

Now the Mullah had a long clean and tidy beard, which is a sign of greatness in the Persian Islamic community. He thought for a moment then said: 'I do not know. I will find out tonight, and then I will let you know.'

So as night came and the Mullah tried to sleep he put his beard over the blanket. After a few minutes his neck became itchy and uncomfortable so he changed the position and put his beard under the blanket. However, that did not help either since it was making him too hot or he couldn't even breathe. In the end he was awake all night, constantly changing the position of the blanket and his beard.

Then he thought to himself and said; I wish I could turn back the clock and stay unaware of my sleeping position.'

The wisdom of this story can be linked to the term called **'NOCEBO EFFECT'**.

Nocebo in Latin means 'I will harm' or 'I shall harm', Not enough research has been done to date on this subject or written about in medical journals, simply because it is not an easy subject to research. Here I would like to mention it as I feel it is an important aspect of the health versus illness subject and needs to be taken into consideration. In his book 'Quantum Healing' Dr. Deepak Chopra briefly mentioned the nocebo effect. And some Japanese researchers also have done experiments with a group of students to monitor the effects this response can have on us.

A nocebo effect is the opposite of placebo effect. In a placebo effect patients have been seen to respond positively, for example, by being given sugar pills and thinking them to be medication for their illness. Some patients have recovered and had a very positive result, but with the nocebo effect, just by being told they have an illness some patients start to get worse and therefore respond negatively.

The reason I mention this nocebo effect is that it looks like in certain circumstances we may be better off not knowing of our conditions since by knowing we can actually harm ourselves. In other words we are our own worst enemy.

For example what is the common knowledge about cancer? Well if we are diagnosed with it our first thought may well be that we are going to die, right? Yet thousands of people have recovered from cancer using various therapies including medical, but yet as soon as one is diagnosed with cancer we can start killing ourselves by our belief.

I vividly remember a lady came into my shop and restlessly began searching amongst the products for something. So I asked her 'Can I help you?' she replied 'No one can help me.' 'Why?' I asked. 'Because a few days ago I have been told I have breast cancer, and I know I will be dead in very short period of time.' I innocently replied, 'Of course you will die, since you are having this kind of attitude.' Then she started to cry. I stayed silent until she became calmer. Then I asked her: 'What has your doctor said about your prognosis?'

(Prognosis: means predicting the likely outcome of a disease based on the condition of the patient and the usual action of the disease).

She told me her doctor said that there was no need to worry, everything would be fine. I said: 'Look your doctor is a responsible and a kind person. Besides your health and wellbeing is your doctor's first priority, so try to follow the advice you are given and also try to seek some support group, of which there are many around, to help in this kind of situation.' Anyhow we had some conversation for a while and as you read you will see and say like me, Lord behold this conversation worked.

I saw her a few times in my shop during that year. I did not see this lady again as I had sold the shop after that. Until one year ago, I was in there picking some items up and in she came. She appeared happy and energetic. I asked her how she was doing, and she replied: 'Never better!' Then after some small talk she said: 'You have no idea how much our conversation that day helped me, I now think being diagnosed with cancer was a major turning point in my life.'

That is almost 12 years ago.

While I was walking to my car, I was thinking of her sentence and the joy in my heart was immeasurable. I thought to myself 'If only we could all respond like this lady'.

I am reminded of a similar case in which another lady was diagnosed with very severe cancer, it had spread all over, her breasts, uterus, fallopian tube and one kidney were affected and consequently removed. Yet she is still alive today after 15 years of being diagnosed. Why? Could it be because of the attitude of both women about their condition, that they decided not to be affected by the nocebo effect?

Let's hope and pray that we never have to face that type of situation, yet if we do let's hope we will have the courage to respond like those ladies did in a time of crisis.

I wish I could say that I have many of those types of stories, but unfortunately they are few. A lot of the time the results of such a diagnosis are so different, yet I believe a high percentage of us could have a positive outcome by choosing to.

You see we 'humans' in times of crises automatically respond negatively. In other words we think of the worst scenario, therefore it is better sometimes to be unaware, and try to only focus on a **WELLNESS** principle and hope all will be fine.

Please do not misunderstand me by thinking that I am suggesting not to do check ups or do blood tests or other precaution testing which are being suggested by your doctor. What I am really saying is this, when we follow wellness principles the chances of being unwell are lessened, therefore there is less chance of serious illnesses. Also our attitude has a major effect on our condition.

I hope I made this point clear for you and you can think and apply this awareness for the betterment of your health.

The nocebo effect is very subtle and no one can really know how they would respond in a time of crises, therefore it is imperative to become strong and try to avoid the circumstances which can cause us to be vulnerable about our health.

As I have said before, many health issues can be dealt with through proper nutrition. A good example of this is the discovery that the lack of Vitamin C is the cause of many of the symptoms mentioned below which are affected by scurvy.

In ancient days lots of people were dying from scurvy. Its effects are characterised by swollen and bleeding gums with loosened teeth, soreness and stiffness of the joints and lower extremities, bleeding under the skin and in deep tissues, slow wound healing, and anemia.

Although accounts of what was probably scurvy are found in ancient writings, the first clear-cut descriptions appear in the records of the medieval Crusades. Later, toward the end of the 15th century, scurvy became the major cause of disability and mortality among sailors on long sea voyages. Not until 1753 was scurvy recognised as related to diet. The concept of deficiency diseases was established for the first time, when the Scottish naval surgeon James Lind showed that scurvy could be cured and prevented by ingestion of the juice of oranges, lemons, or limes.

In modern times, full-blown cases of vitamin C deficiency have become relatively rare; in the United States, they may still be seen in isolated elderly adults, usually men whose diet is limited to foods lacking in vitamin C, and in infants fed reconstituted milk or milk substitutes without a vitamin C or orange juice supplement. Symptoms peculiar to infantile scurvy (Barlow's disease) include swelling of the lower extremities, pain upon flexing them, and lesions of the growing bones.

Administration of vitamin C is the specific therapy for scurvy. Even in cases of severe deficiency, a daily dose of 100 milligrams for adults or 10 to 25 milligrams for infants and children, accompanied by a normal diet, commonly produces a cure within several days. This very simple information has saved thousands of lives since its discovery.

As we saw in, **The Story of a Mullah and His Beard,** informing ourselves sometimes can bring about anxiety and restlessness. So it is important to free your mind from worrying knowledge and concentrate on the positive and wellness. You see the reason I am spending so much time on this issue is because of its importance in our daily life. Even sometimes just a simple question can bring anxiety and trigger the **'NOCEBO EFFECT'**.

So let me finish this subject with this incident.

Although, this incident happened many years ago, yet I am embarrassed to remember the immaturity of my question to one of my clients.

A lady came to me, complaining of unusually severe tiredness. She was over thirty years old, a single girl who had been disappointed in love. She also had all the other symptoms of Multiple Sclerosis.

I asked her if she had ever been diagnosed with having MS.

She replied with a look of fear in her face. 'No! Why do you ask this question?'

Well my next comment made the situation even worse. I said, 'Because you have some symptoms which are common to MS sufferers.' Then immediately I said, 'But do not worry everything will be fine.'

The more I tried to comfort her the worse the situation got. It was like a small hole in the sand – the more you fiddle with it the bigger the hole becomes.

I know that some physicians would be proud of making that kind of diagnosis without a blood test. Even when I discussed this case with a female colleague she admired me for noticing the condition so swiftly. The girl was later diagnosed as having MS but she never came back to me because she experienced that deep fear as a result of my ineptitude. Now even today I am still confused. Did she develop MS because I saw the similarities of her condition with MS sufferers or did she already have that condition in her? It is hard to say, isn't it?

I fully sympathise with all allopathic physicians who have a large amount of knowledge and who can easily fall into such traps of this kind of situation. Even by a mere facial expression any physician could make a patient worry. You see when we know something is wrong it is very difficult to pretend that everything is O.K. I hope I am making sense.

However, I will talk about the whole subject of nutrition later in its own section. So let's go back and finish what we were saying. But maybe I am getting much too serious now. So let's have a little story – maybe a funny one entitled:

THE STORY OF A MAN WITH DRY BREAD.

One day in Persia a man arrived at a special type of restaurant which is so prevalent in **RASHT** my home town in north-east Persia. These types of restaurants are only open in the early morning and specialise in cooking '**AHSH**' or '**HALEEM**', which in the West would be similar to soup or porridge, but the taste and ingredients are very different. The restaurant is set up in such a way so it can serve indoors or outdoors. A big pot of the soup is on display at the opening to tempt one, as the aroma wafts onto the street and invites one in to purchase some.

Anyway this is the story of a man who arrived at the restaurant. He approached the owner and said to him, I have some dry bread and wondered if you would be so kind and give me some '**AHSH**' for free? Since I am very hungry and have travelled a long distance and have no money to pay for a bowl of ahsh. The owner refused and told the man to go away. The man stood there and was puzzled as to what to do, then he had a great idea. He stood beside the big pot and held his dry bread above the pot as the steam of the delicious soup was evaporating, so his bread became moistened and tasted relatively pleasant.

As he finished and was ready to leave, the owner of the restaurant called to him: 'Where are you going? You need to pay me.'

The man replied: 'Pay you for what?'

With a surprised look on his face, the owner said :'For the steam of the soup which you used'.

The man said: 'My friend, you are the meanest person I have ever met in my life. The steam of the soup is going to waste anyway, how can you be that mean to ask me to pay for it.'

The owner said: 'The steam of the soup is a part of my business. If

Illness and Welllness – The Connections

everybody who arrived here and used only the steam and didn't pay me, I would soon be poor like you'

So the argument continued on until they decided to go to court to obtain a just ruling.

The wise judge listened to the complete story and then delivered his verdict, saying to the restaurant owner: 'In truth, you are right. You need to be paid the correct price of the steam of your soup. So please tell me how much do you want for it?'

The owner of the restaurant mentioned some amount in Persian currency of the time, whereupon the judge put his hand into his pocket and took out the amount requested. He then dropped the coins to the ground and as they fell they made a jingling sound.

So the judge said to the owner: 'You can take the jingling sound of the money as payment for the steam of your soup.'

I am not entirely sure if you will have enjoyed this story, but my understanding of it is this: There are times when some of us are like the characters in that story. Sometimes we may act like that poor man in order to survive with as little as that steam, then other times behave like the owner of the restaurant and even sometimes like the wise judge. I feel parents who have two children or more would appreciate this story for it illustrates how at times they need to be as wise as the judge in loving their children fairly and equally.

Please promise me that you will act like that wise judge when I tell you the next story. In fact the above story has been in preparation for the next one.

There is another thought right now going through my mind which if I share it with you I would be afraid that you would throw away the book and would think I had lost my mind altogether. You know what? I am actually going to share it with you. I feel so close to you since you have read this much of the book. In fact I feel by now we kind of know each other and hopefully have become friends. I feel like this with you! I hope you feel close to me too.

Anyway the other thought is this: some of the giant pharmaceutical companies sometimes dismiss the findings of scientists who have made discoveries which suggest other forms of medicine or therapies might have a better effect on the health and wellbeing of the public than modern medical treatments. You and I as the public deserve to know these findings.

I feel their action is like the owner of the restaurant who can't even give away the steam of his soup. The point which I am referring to is the use of natural and alternative medicine. The interest by the public in alternative medicine is a fraction of our health care, and the percentage of sales of natural and alternative medicine is negligible in comparison to what pharmaceuticals earn annually through sales of prescribed medicine. As God is my witness I have no problem with that, I hope they earn more next year, but with one difference, and that is if they can provide us with better satisfactory results than at present, and I hope we will have less and less sick people in our society.

I am aware of how hard it is to mention any new health discovery which appears to be contradictory to the present medical establishment, without some people feeling offended particularly some pharmacists, doctors or some members of the public whose life has been saved or is dependent on the use of medicine. No doubt they are saving lives daily, but this does not mean everything they do is right. My evaluation measurement is based on the result. If we are having more and more people who are sick then we must look around to see if we can change our way of thinking. You know I feel this subject is like one of those holes in the sand which I mentioned before, the more I try to fix it the bigger the hole becomes.

Anyhow the purpose of me mentioning the following is to make you aware of the large amounts of discoveries which if followed through properly, have possibilities of having a very different outcome in the health care system.

Let's hope that will happen soon.

You know what? I am actually going to tell you one of the stories which were for some 30 years pushed aside, but as we say in Persia:

TIME WILL CORRECT THE INCORRECT CIRCUMSTANCES

Illness and Welllness – The Connections

As you read I hope you will agree with me that this Persian saying was right in relation to this story which I am going to tell you now. An innocent pathologist lost 30 years of his career life due to one of his discoveries on homocysteine.

How many of us believe it when we are told the sentence below about cholesterol?

High cholesterol is the cause of heart attacks and stroke.

Well, one man thought differently, it took him more then 30 years to prove this scientifically.

I can guess what you may be thinking about this sentence and maybe saying to yourself. *He can't be serious?*

So let's find out shall we. I call this:

THE STORY OF HOMOCYSTEINE
This story comes from the understanding I have gained from reading a book by Dr Kilmer McCully entitled *The Homocysteine Revolutions* – I am sharing with you the short version of it.

It does not begin with the words 'Once upon a time' because it is a story of the present and I shall begin simply by asking: How many of us have heard that high cholesterol is the main cause of heart disease and stroke? Well I myself believed this to be true almost up to the year 2000. We have been told this for almost three decades, and billions are being made by the companies who produce/sell these cholesterol-reducing drugs. Apparently Dr Kilmer McCully with his genius mind wasn't happy with what he was seeing with his own eyes; therefore he researched, studied and followed these findings for 30 years of his life, in order to bring the truth out about the issue of cholesterol.

Well I will give you some facts to start with.

Apparently most people, who have a heart attack, actually have a normal cholesterol level.

Also, most people with high cholesterol have hearts that are in good shape.

Please remember I said 'most people' not 'all people' because there are exceptions. Besides the issue of cholesterol is so complex, that not only is it hard to explain it is even harder to understand. But if we ask ourselves a simple question, which is this, when there is an over amount of a substance in our body, would it be sensible for us to reduce the consumption of foods which contain a lot of that substance in order to overcome the problem? Yes it would. Yet we go and purchase medicine to reduce the amount of that substance.

(Note: for more information and clarifications on the issue of fat and cholesterol you can read a book by **Uffe Ravnskov MD** called '**The Cholesterol Myths**'.)

You see, snow did not bring winter; it was winter which brought snow. High cholesterol is the by-product of poor nutrition or poor diet. By reducing cholesterol via medication we do not solve the problem of poor diet, and poor nutrition, and we only sell to the poor victim of high cholesterol a product with unpleasant side effects. This idea is becoming more and more evident amongst a genuine and caring medical community. Also I would like to predict something here which I believe will bear its fruits within 2 to 5 years, and that is;

ALL THE CHOLESTEROL REDUCING PRODUCTS WILL BE REMOVED FROM THE MARKET FOR TWO REASONS: THE UNPLEASANT AND UNACCEPTABLE SIDE EFFECTS

It does not solve the original problem in the first place.

What is **HOMOCYSTEINE** anyway? In fact its own story is an interesting one.

Doctor Kilmer McCully the author mentioned above was a promising pathologist and researcher who graduated from Harvard Medical School in the mid-1960s. Dr. McCully enjoyed studies that involved the connection of biochemistry with disease. His reputation was strong, and he soon landed prestigious positions as an Associate Pathologist at Massachusetts General Hospital and as an Assistant Professor of Pathology at Harvard Medical School.

So let's see what happened to him and his reputation. Early in Dr. McCully's career, he became interested in a disease called

HOMOCYSTINURIA. This disease presented itself in children who had a genetic defect that kept them from breaking down an essential amino acid called **METHIONINE**. These children showed a tremendous build-up of a by-product called **HOMOCYSTEINE**. McCully reviewed two separate cases involving young boys with this defect who died of heart attacks. This was quite amazing since both of these boys were not even eight years old. When he examined the boys' pathology slides, he discovered that the damage to the arteries was eerily similar to that of an elderly man who had severe hardening of the arteries, as in atherosclerosis.

This led Dr. McCully to wonder whether mild to moderate elevations of **HOMOCYSTEINE** that were present over a lifetime could be a cause of heart attacks and strokes in the average patient. As seen previously in the case of the two boys, **HOMOCYSTEINE** is an intermediate by-product that we produce when our bodies metabolise or break down the essential amino acid **METHIONINE**.

METHIONINE is found in large quantities in our meats, eggs, milk, cheese, white flour, canned foods, and highly processed foods. Our bodies need **METHIONINE** to survive. However, as you can see from the list of foods that contain large quantities of this nutrient, people of the Western world have plenty of it in their diet. **CYSTEINE** and **METHIONINE** are benign products and are not harmful to us in any way. But here is the catch: the enzymes needed to break down **HOMOCYSTEINE** into cysteine or back to **METHIONINE** need folic acid, B12, B6 and also some B3 vitamins to do their job.

If we are deficient in these nutrients, the levels of **HOMOCYSTEINE** in the blood begin to rise. So why haven't we heard this before?

BINGO! Here is the answer: because nobody can patent the green vegetables like cabbages or spinach and put them exclusively under their corporate name. So they are not interested in educating us about it.

If you take the above mentioned vitamins through your daily diet, eating plenty of green-leaved vegetables, like cabbage, spinach and wholegrain foods or organically grown supplements, then the level of your homocysteine declines and you will not suffer from hardening of the arteries. Nor will you have problems with your heart. It is very important for us to understand this, since two out of every three deaths are associated with some form of heart disorder.

So why aren't we told the truth? Well this is up to each of us to find out just like I did. You see nobody posted information to my house. I went and I found out for myself. Now you are perhaps in your own home reading these facts for the first time. The question is what are you going to do with this information?

I chose this story from amongst many other scientific findings I have researched because of the vast proportions of health budgets which are today being wasted on reducing cholesterol and I am no longer happy to remain quiet and keep my mouth closed on this subject. The other significant findings I tracked down include: Professor John Beards' *Trophoblasti* **THESIS OF CANCER** (*Edinburgh University*) and Dr.Fereydoon Batmanghelidj's **WATER CURE THESIS** as well as Andrew Wyllie's findings on **APOPTOSIS,** Dr.Patch Adams **'GESUNDHEIT' LAUGHING CLINICS** and Dr Deepak Chopra's work on **QUANTUM HEALING.** The full list is endless and I will refer to some of these topics in more detail in an Appendix about outstanding healers past and present that appears at the end of this book.

But don't worry; the news is not all bad! We have enough good news in this slim volume to keep you happy for the rest of your life. So let's continue now by focussing really closely in the following chapters on **WELLNESS.** That is a good place to put our spotlight – in fact the very best of places – and in the next few pages I intend to explore with you in detail the **FOUR GOLDEN PRINCIPLES OF GOOD HEALTH AND WELLBEING** outlined very briefly indeed near the front of this book. They combine modern science with my own years of complementary health practice experience in Ireland and academic wisdom from Ancient Persia. These four fundamental principles are so simple that they will not have any ill effects on anybody – no matter whether you are on a diet or taking prescribed medicine or are observing any particular food restrictions for religious or other reasons.

You can follow these simple principles and apply them easily in your daily life, step by step. One day you will possibly be teaching others how to follow them. They are so simple that you can apply them and teach them to others from the very first day that you discover them – if you so choose. It is up to you because in essence **WELLNESS** is simply a matter of achieving equilibrium between physical, mental, and emotional being and developing the ability to cope with our environment

Finally I would like to finish this chapter with an important quotation, which took me many years to understand and accept. It encapsulates very succinctly the powerful idea that in the end our wellbeing is simply in our own hands. The quotation says:

There is no such thing as an incurable disease, there are only incurable people.

Wellness Can Be Summed Up In One Word – HARMONY

CHAPTER SEVEN

WELLNESS – HOW I LOVE THAT TERM!

What a beautiful term is **WELLNESS**. I really love it. It is like music to my ears. Have you ever truly thought of the idea of being well and healthy? It may even appear to some as impossible to achieve. You will possibly be surprised when you see how easy it is in reality to achieve health and wellness.

If your natural response is '**I would never be able to do it**', you need to remember that never is a very long time. I mean, how would you respond to serious news about your health tomorrow or next year? You never know! Wouldn't you agree? Of course you would.

So why not learn healthy habits? It may be useful come the rainy day – as any Irish person may say. But first let's define the words health and wellness. To me Wellness is a wonderful state – like beautiful spontaneous poetry.

WELLNESS IS BEING HAPPY WITH EVERYTHING AROUND US, EVERYTHING ABOUT US, BEING ABLE TO COPE WITH OUR WORK, FAMILY, FRIENDS, ECONOMY, ENVIRONMENT, WELLNESS IS MAINTAINING A BALANCE BETWEEN WHAT WE LOVE AND WHAT WE STRIVE FOR, BETWEEN WHO WE ARE AND WHO WE WANT TO BECOME; INDEED WELLNESS CAN BE SUMMED UP IN ONE WORD: HARMONY

I did not mean to write that definition as a poem, it just turned into one on its own. And after that tiny lyrical flight of fancy, let me tell you another little story. This story unlike most of the previous ones does not really have a name; it is just a true account of something that happened recently. It can perhaps best be called:

A STORY WITHOUT A NAME

In fact it happened just a few weeks ago and it was a very windy and rainy day. I was at home and had a Persian friend visiting me. He was just back from Persia, and we were having a late and leisurely breakfast. After breakfast I suggested we go for a little walk. Well I had better tell you that we are blessed having a beautiful house in very friendly countryside on the top of a hill surrounded by lush green fields. The wind howled as I opened the front door and was so strong it almost blew it back in my face. We were dressed in outdoor gear, hats, coats, boots, gloves, the lot, I tell you this so you may get a picture of how challenging this wind was. High on top of one of our trees there is a crow's nest and it was taking a battering from the wind.

'Look,' I said to my friend, 'it almost looks as if the wind and rain are trying to destroy the poor crow's nest.'

But strangely enough the crows had such a perfect nest, that in all the years we had lived there, the wind and rain have never harmed it. But now the scene was so disturbing that I found it difficult to watch. I wanted to bring the crows inside to keep them warm, safe and dry until the wind had gone. But that would have been interfering with nature, wouldn't it?

Now here is the point that I wish to make. Nature is harmony. That means it is neither **RIGHT** nor **WRONG**. But we humans almost always insist on making things 'right' from our point of view don't we? And this is possibly the cause of a lot of disharmony in our societies.

Imagine if there was a Crow's Committee or Crow's Union. It might well riot or strike about the cruelty of the wind and rain. We might have a Crow TV Channel talking and squawking about how much damage has been done by the wind. They might even have believed that the wind had some kind of WMD – weapons of mass destruction!

Welllness – How I Love That Term!

As crazy as this may sound, it is, strangely enough, what we humans do. So if you want to be healthy and well all the time, try learning about **HARMONY.** You may be surprised at the joy it will bring to your life. You will see that all events in your daily life are for your highest good.

In over 20 years of experience, by learning, practising complementary health care and from my clinical observations, I have learned the importance of four golden principles which essentially constitute **HEALTH** and **WELLNESS.**

So without further ado let's find out what those four principles are in detail – and how we can apply them in our daily life.

The Very Greatest
Secret of Your Life
Is To Realise
Every Minute of Every Day
What is RIGHT About It
Rather Than
What is WRONG With It

CHAPTER EIGHT

GOLDEN PRINCIPLE NUMBER ONE

BE GRATEFUL

Being grateful is very different from positive thinking. That does not mean I undervalue positive thinking in any way. The good effects of positive thinking are endless and enormous and should not by any means be underestimated. Yet for me the true essence of being grateful is expressed best in the following phrase, which I have conjured up after a lot of thought:

BEING GRATEFUL REALLY MEANS TO BE ABLE TO SAY A PRAYER WITHOUT USING WORDS.

However, the aspect of being grateful that I would like to talk about first here is based on the quotation which I have placed at the beginning of this chapter. For me this comes under the heading of 'unfolding the secrets of life.' And I feel it will bear repetition:

The Greatest Secret of our Life is, to realise in every moment what is, **RIGHT** *about it, rather than, what is* **WRONG** *with it.*

This principle may appear to be very simple and elementary – yet nonetheless it is arguably the most important principle of health that I know. You see with the advancement of today's modern health technology, we can purchase a lot of things to correct our health and physical shortcomings, but we can't buy the principle of **BEING GRATEFUL**.

For example, if we are not happy with the shape of our bodies, our faces or the shape and size of our breasts we can go, provided we have sufficient money, to have surgery to change ourselves to some extent to whatever size and shape we desire. Or we can have a heart transplant or a kidney or liver transplant, which in truth are like miracles. But no matter how poor or rich we are, no matter how healthy or unhealthy we are, no matter how highly important an individual we may be, we cannot purchase a **GOOD ATTITUDE**.

We have to learn that for ourselves and try to apply it in our life. We can make all the excuses under the sun about our circumstances but there is really only one person who is responsible for our attitude – and that is ourselves, nobody else.

I love this line by Pat Mesiti:

> **'If someone spits on you, they do not injure your dignity or honour, all they do is to make you a little wet.'**

Pat Mesiti is a motivational speaker who works in Australia and New Zealand and has produced some remarkable results in his field of specialisation. He is best known for his work with youth groups and he has helped thousands of disadvantaged and disturbed young people to overcome their life challenges.

How many times have we heard the story of a person with great self-belief who by controlling his or her mind recovers from some seemingly fatal illness as a result? Well now new scientific research can demonstrate the overwhelming power of this principle and prove conclusively why we need to apply this principle in our life. And what is the secret? In just one word it is: **DOPAMINE**

Yes that's right, Dopamine. It is a relatively simple chemical substance, a hormone in fact. And whenever we choose to be grateful, it is now known that we actually secrete this hormone Dopamine in our own body.

When we enjoy life, for whatever reason, when we give pleasure to our body by eating delicious food, dancing or lovemaking, or by having any other pleasing, enjoyable or pleasant experience, then our brain will grant us a reward and release this hormone in our bodies. Also we can achieve similar effects through simple mental activity.

For example if we just enjoy listening to birds singing or seeing the moon rise or the sun setting, if we gaze happily at the horizon out to sea and appreciate life in any or every way in our surroundings, we are instantly rewarded by our brain with an inner secretion of these miracle hormones. Isn't that an extraordinary truth? What could be easier? It is like having our own chemist shop or pharmacy inside us isn't it, ready to serve us the perfect safe prescription for all our needs – and without any negative side effects.

Let's now see what this means scientifically and how we can apply this knowledge best in our daily lives. Rather than giving you a long medical text book version of the background to this information, which might leave you needing further clarification, I am going to tell you my version of it.

DOPAMINE is in the simplest terms a hormone that acts as a neurotransmitter or chemical transmitter for our cells. This means it makes the cells wake up and move and get on efficiently with the jobs they were designed to do. Deficiency of this hormone can cause schizophrenia, Parkinson's disease and manic depression.

So exactly where do we obtain this hormone? As I said earlier effectively in our own inner private pharmacy that has got a sign saying **BRAIN** over its 'shop front'. If we want to be even more accurate, we should say the glands – and the King of All the Glands is the **PITUITARY** that is situated in our brain.

Our capability to produce good hormones internally, however, is not limited to Dopamine. The pituitary gland itself, the King Gland or Master Gland, is like a wise person sitting quietly in a room who knows everything that is going on. Yet the King has several other important royal supporters in the form of other glands where they can produce many other hormones that also create very positive outcomes in our body. It really is up to us whether we create them or not – and now we know about this, what is to stop us doing it? Nothing at all! If we are prepared to just make the effort.

So I will tell you briefly here about a few more of these very helpful substances. First let's look at Serotonin, then Endorphins and finally Melatonin.

SEROTONIN or 5-HTP (5-HYDROXYTRYPTAMINE) is another neurotransmitter that acts positively to stimulate our cells. It is concentrated in certain areas of the brain, especially the midbrain and the **HYPOTHALAMUS** gland and changes in its concentration are associated with mood swings. Some cases of mental depression are apparently caused by reduced quantities or reduced activity of Serotonin in the brain.

ENDORPHINS are substances working throughout the whole nervous system and they are composed of amino acids. They are made by the **PITUITARY** gland and act on the nervous system to reduce pain. They produce similar effects to morphine and there is strong evidence that endorphins are connected with what are called the 'pleasure centers' in our brain.

MELATONIN is a hormone and in humans it seems to play an important role in the regulation of our sleep cycles. Melatonin is secreted by the **PINEAL** gland, a tiny endocrine gland situated at the centre of the brain. Melatonin was discovered in 1958 by American physician Aaron B. Lerner and his colleagues at Yale University School of Medicine. A derivative of the amino acid, tryptophan, Melatonin is produced in humans, other mammals, birds, reptiles, and amphibians.

So that is a very short lesson about a few of our own self-produced 'wonder substances.' I trust it will help you realise that we have amazing resources at our disposal inside ourselves. Isn't it strange that we spend millions buying drugs in the hope of making ourselves feel better, yet we can have the best and most useful substances that our own bodies can produce completely free of charge.

So now I guess you are going to ask me: Well, how exactly do we do it? My answer is this: if you read the next few lines objectively, I believe eighty per cent of your life can become happy. So I will quickly give you a few examples of how these 'happy hormones' can be produced by your own body. And you can start straight away.

Example No 1: Tomorrow morning when you wake up you have two choices. You can say either:

"**Good morning, God, thank you for another day!**"

Or you can say:

"**Good God, it's morning. Not another day!**"

Golden Principle Number One

So you see from those two choices that the key to whether you are happy or sad in truth is in your own hands. Well to be more accurate it is actually in your head well, all right to be absolutely correct it is in your mind. But be that as it may, nobody else is responsible for your happiness, except you…And that choice you make as you wake up will either trigger good chemical responses in your body or not. It's entirely up to you. Here is another example:

Example No 2: Imagine you go out shopping, and on your way back it suddenly starts raining heavily and by the time you get to your transport vehicle you are absolutely soaked. You could say;

"Thanks to God! I have some form of transport!"

Or you can say:

"Damn it! What a miserable day!"

In general terms we talk negatively to others and ourselves all the time, without realising the adverse effect it has on our own health. It is something we might guard against more carefully if we remembered how this affects things inside our bodies, and the substances we secrete or do not secrete as a result. So it is time isn't it, to wise up? Here are some positive and negative examples of this:

On Saturdays traffic is very **BAD** in our city . . . **NEGATIVE** statement
On Saturdays traffic is very busy in our city . . . . **POSITIVE** statement

You might be asked: Would you like an appointment on Friday?

No, Friday is a very **BAD** day for me . . . . **NEGATIVE**
No, Friday is not a suitable day for me . . . . **POSITIVE**

Or you might be telling somebody about where you live:

Our house is located after that very **BAD** bend . . . . **NEGATIVE**
Our house is located after that sharp bend . . . . **POSITIVE**

On another occasion, you might find yourself saying:

I am dying to get home . . . . **NEGATIVE**
I am looking forward to getting home . . . . **POSITIVE**

Then there is the most common example of all:

I am very tired .... **This is a very NEGATIVE statement**

Here are a few **positive** ways of saying it:

> I would love to get some sleep.
> I am going to enjoy my sleep tonight.
> My body will benefit greatly from some rest tonight.

And so on and so forth...You can, I am sure, easily add quite a few examples of your own and do please feel free to do so...From this it can be seen that all of our daily conversations need to be adjusted gradually from negative to positive. If you want that 'happy pharmacy' of yours inside you to stay open twenty-four hours a day, these are some of the keys that can help you make it happen.

Now this does not mean that negative things never happen in your life. But it does mean that you can have a positive attitude to correct them. I risk repeating myself here, but perhaps intelligent repetition can be the way we learn important lessons. You simply have to come to terms with the fact that you and you alone are in the driver's seat. You make the decisions about your life and your health, nobody else!

Again the last but not the least statement is: **THE CHOICE IS YOURS!**

* * * * * * * *

In fairness I wish to say: Of course I do not know about your life and it may well be that you have some heavy challenges going on right now. But I can promise you, if you try to find something that is **RIGHT** about your life, a great deal can quickly change.

You could start like this:

> **"I am so glad that I have eyes and can see. Or, I am educated and can read."**

This in itself will be a very good start. But of course we all have our own versions of the truth. Like an interesting lady who comes to me once or twice a year and whenever she is in trouble. She has been involved in

Golden Principle Number One

several relationships and each time ends up with a married man who is in the process of getting separated. She is good looking and very young and it puzzles me the perception she has about herself and the types of relationships that she gets involved in.

More than once I have asked her: 'Why don't you get involved with single men?'

And she replies: 'Where are there any single men? I can't find any.'

And this is almost over a ten-year period. Strangely I know a few men and women who find themselves in this kind of situation. They are not looking at what is right in their life, they keep on doing something that they do not really want to. This is because they do not change their way of thinking and only see their lives from one perspective.

While we are on this subject, let me tell you something interesting about being able to see.

A few months ago my eldest daughter Emily and I went for a walk. It was night time and there was a beautiful, dark blue moonlit sky above us spangled with lots of stars. I said to my daughter: 'Look, Em,' and pointed to the moon as it shone through a tree that was leafless because of the winter season. The moon was truly beautiful that night and from time to time was being covered by light clouds.

Emily said: 'My God! That is so beautiful. It is like watching a movie.'

Next morning I woke up and went for a walk. This time my little girl Ruth, who is twelve years old, came along. It was just before sunrise. The moon was still visible and so big like the sun, but of course on the opposite side of the sky to the sun. Looking up at it, Ruth said: 'WOW! This is so wonderful! I never saw the moon that big before.'

Those were truly treasured moments that I shared a few hours apart with my two daughters. It reminded me that there is so much beauty around us that is always there for us, free of charge. But so often we are so deeply engaged with our lives that we actually forget the simplest and most wonderful ways of living.

But there is a particular reason beyond that why I am telling you this story at this point in the book. You see, a few months prior to that night I was interviewed by our local radio station about health matters and my approach to them and this interview generated a lot of interest in our area. As a result a young man accidentally heard my name and came to see me. He was around twenty years old but was ninety-seven per cent blind.

It turned out he had a disease called, **LHON** which stands for *Leber Hereditary Optic Neuropathy*. It is a hereditary and genetic disorder and in his case he had it because his Mum and Dad's genes were not compatible to each other. As a result when such people have children there is a possibility of them developing this disease. As it happens he is the second child in his family who is affected in this way and is going blind.

I found myself thinking: If he was my child, how could I show him the beautiful moon and the sunset and all the other wonders of nature's scenery? I suppose the point I am trying to make is this: It is not his fault that his Mum and Dad fell in love and got married and as a result he is losing his sight. But look at us! Yes you and me and many others who can see! We have been given the privilege of being able to see and read. And how many times do we say a word of appreciation for this gift?

If that would happen to me, how much would I be prepared to pay in order to have my eyesight returned? How much would you pay? But now, because we have it for free, most of us take it for granted and forget to appreciate the value of it. Too often we find other things wrong with our life that we can complain about.

Possibly that young man has to find out what life has in store for him. Sometimes with that kind of physical challenge people do things which can be considered remarkable and make better lives for thousands of others if they can find the purpose of their challenge. Like Blair Hill, son of Napoleon Hill (author of the famous book *Think and Grown Rich*) who was born with no physical sign of ears and the family doctor admitted that the child might be deaf and mute for life.

But having inherited a powerful mind from his father, Blair persisted in seeking solutions and in the end, not only did he find a solution for his own hearing impairment he found solutions for thousands of others too. He started by assisting hearing aid manufacturers to re-design and improve their products.

When he could hear with the aid of their hearing instruments, then it turned out that many other deaf people could hear with these products too. So Blair Hill turned his severe disadvantage to good account, improved his own life and helped others like himself in the process. This is a very short version of their story; the whole tale is to be found in Napoleon Hill's inspirational book **Think and Grow Rich.** It is a powerful book, and at times when I feel challenged in my life, I have learned to look at the challenge and to find the hidden opportunity within it.

Nonetheless, I do feel that the ability to see and enjoy the beauty of our surroundings is truly a precious gift of life.

When contemplating what gifts there are to be grateful for, I feel I have to say, that I can promise you, if you are living in the Western world, there are many things for which it is right to feel grateful. And if your answer is: 'But still my life is so difficult' – and this may indeed be true – then I think the question you must ask yourself is:

WHAT CAN I LEARN FROM THESE CIRCUMSTANCES IN WHICH I FIND MYSELF?

You know it is like the story of a person who was wondering why he receives a letter every six months regarding his driving test. Well the simple answer is he receives the letter because he has not passed the driving test yet. You see there is nothing magical about people who are healthy all the time. They are healthy because their attitude and lifestyle choices keep them healthy.

While on this subject I feel moved to admit that I can talk a lot about this First Golden Principle. In fact it's true to say that a twenty-five per cent success rate on each of the Four Principles will ensure total optimal health for any person. In my own case I will confess I need to apply this one almost eighty per cent of the time to succeed. Personally I find the other Three Golden Principles easier to follow than the first and wish for the day when I can find this one as easy to apply without effort.

Many years ago I taught myself a 'habit' designed to make it easier to apply this First Principle regularly in my life. This is it: Every morning when I wake up I go for a little walk around the house and along the country road. I purposely thank God for twelve things that are **RIGHT** about my life and twelve gifts that I am receiving daily. Honestly some time it is so hard even to think of one but I force myself to say it and by the time I am back from my walk I am almost a different person. It is like I have opened up my own little internal 'happy pharmacy' and received all the free, happy medications in exact proportions.

Here is another affirmation you may find helpful to say daily in order to make yourself feel great:

**I AM LIVING IN A WONDERFUL PRESENT,
WALKING TOWARDS A BEAUTIFUL FUTURE,
LETTING GO OF THE PAST WITH LOVE,
I FEEL YOUNG AGAIN!!!**

To close, I wish to bless this chapter with a prayer from the book, **Persian Hidden Words** which was revealed by **BAHA'ULLAH,** the founder of the **BAHA'I** faith. I visit this prayer every day alongside my other daily prayers. I feel anyone who reaches the stations that are mentioned in **Persian Hidden Words** can truly be considered as a person who has inner contentment and the ability to receive the joyful pleasures of life. The prayer, which I will place alone on the next page, goes like this:

O COMPANION OF MY THRONE!

Hear no evil, and see no evil, abase not thyself, neither sigh nor weep. Speak no evil, that thou mayest not hear it spoken unto thee, and magnify not the faults of others that thine own faults may not appear great; and wish not the abasement of anyone, that thine own abasement be not exposed. Live then the days of thy life, that are less than a fleeting moment, with thy mind stainless, thy heart unsullied, thy thoughts pure, and thy nature sanctified, so that, free and content, thou mayest put away this mortal frame, and repair unto the mystic paradise and abide in the eternal kingdom for evermore.

You Are Not
SICK
You Are
THIRSTY

CHAPTER NINE

GOLDEN PRINCIPLE NUMBER TWO

DRINK ENOUGH WATER

At this moment what I would ask you to do, is to put the book down and close your eyes and focus your thoughts upon the importance of water in your surroundings and in your life. Visualise what it would be like if there was not enough water available to you.

It is frightening, isn't it?

Every cell, tissue, and organ in our body needs water to survive and function properly. For hygiene and for cleaning most things, the first substance we need is water. We wash our clothes, our bodies, our cars and our dishes. It would be sensible to say that we need to wash our inner selves with water too.

Would you believe that I paused for a few days when I got to this chapter, I could not get my mind to settle and start to write about water. There is so much to be said about water that I didn't know where to start. Already there is so much written about water, from the ability of water to retain memory, to the scientific and biological reason that we need to drink it; from getting a hexagon picture of the structure of frozen water, to seeing that water has a great message within it that is there to sustain our health.

Also I have already come across several books written about every angle that you can imagine about water and its capability to dramatically change our life, including its effects on our emotional behaviour. Please refer to the Appendix in this book for a list of books about water.

You see, sometimes, when so much has been said about a subject, it can be challenging to say something which is relatively new and useful. Therefore I have decided to write simple and essential information about the importance of drinking water daily, and other useful information that you need to know about the ways in which water affects our health.

For example how much water is the correct amount to drink? When should we drink water? Do some need more water than others? What is the importance of bottled water, jug filtering system, distillations, compressed block technology with UV light?

You know if I would tell you my honest feelings about the importance of drinking water for our body, it would be very brief.

Drink 2 to 3 litres of PURE, CLEAN, CLEAR, **WATER** everyday. When I am saying 2 to 3 litres of water, I mean only water, nothing else. In other words I do not mean tea, coffee, soft drinks or beverages. I mean only undiluted PURE, CLEAN, CLEAR water. You see water is the simplest substance in the world, so when we add other things to it, we break its structure, therefore it cannot be as effective as it is when pure.

Did you know that many diseases like Asthma, allergies, migraine headaches, irritable bowel syndrome, stomach ulcer and so on and so forth, can be prevented by water alone?

Water is the only substance that we cannot keep too much of in our body system. This is different from other substances. Too much **SUGAR** in our bodies can cause **diabetes**. Too much **SALT** can cause **atherosclerosis** which refers to the hardening of the **arteries**. Too much **FAT** can cause all kinds of **heart disease**. Instead, water creates movement and this is one of the conditions that we need in order to be at a stage of well being, because the movement of water on its way to our elimination organs collects toxins from our body and gives a sensation of lightness.

You might be thinking that **fluid retention** means that there is too much water in our body system. But my answer is **NO,** it is not, because fluid retention means that there is too much water in the body's outer cells. In fact fluid retention is actually the symptoms of dehydration. Drugs which are taken to help that condition have so far not offered any long term improvements.

Finally, please note that I said 'prevented' not 'cured' three paragraphs earlier, since prevention can stop them accruing in the first place. That is why I chose to start this chapter with the quotation:

YOU ARE NOT SICK YOU ARE THIRSTY.

What a true and powerful statement. The first person to write it was, Dr. FEREYDOON BATMANGHELIDJ who is known as Dr.B for short. A short account of his theories and his life story is given in an Appendix to this book.

In early 1990 the University of Georgia in U.S.A. did a study on diseased cells, and compared them to healthy cells. The results showed that the only difference between them was, the healthy cell had structured water and the diseased cell had unstructured water.

So let me explain about structured and unstructured water. Unless it moves all the time water becomes unstructured then dead or stagnant. Water ideally needs to fall, particularly from a height, which makes it much more alive, since it collects more oxygen on its way down.

Have you noticed that moving water such as seen in rivers is clearer looking than the still water in lakes? The reason for all of this is the structure of the water. When water has movement and particularly in water falls, the water cluster is in a condition where its molecular structure is described as having a 'right circular radial force'. Then as it is pumped through pipes or processed to create beverages, water's structure is converted to a molecular chain structure with a 'left circular radial force'.

You can help to reverse this to a small degree by filling up a one or two litre jug size with water, and then stir the water vigorously in an anti-clockwise direction for a few seconds, then do it clockwise for a few more seconds, and repeat this a few times. Then leave the water to settle for one hour or more, so that the water can stay free and some of the water cluster structure can return to its original condition. Let me give you some further tips:

- If possible do not drink water which has been left around, either in or out of the fridge for more than seven days.

- Please note there are products on the market which brings back the water cluster to its original state. One kind that I know of is called a **DRINK HARMONISER** but this system does not remove the chemicals from water.

- **The best time** for drinking water is from sun rise to sun set; since the particles from the sun called 'photons', or Light Quantum activates the components of the cells in our body, when we have enough water in our system it prevents the accumulation of toxic waste.

- **The easiest way** to drink water is, two glasses every hour. This will create a habit and bring about a natural rhythm of thirst, gradually.

- Water is good for us, if it is **good water**.

- **Purification** of our drinking water has to be the first health action that we take.

- **The fountain of youth** comes from our tap, in our kitchen, when we make sure it has been purified.

- **70 % of our body is water**, so the question we need to ask, is 70 % of our intake water?

- **Chlorine** is at this moment the most affective way of eliminating impurities in our drinking water in cities and counties, it is **not essential for our inner organism**.

- **Water is an empty substance.** It has the capacity to carry almost every thing with it, including VOCs otherwise known as volatile organic compounds, and also heavy metals like lead and mercury. These are not essential in our drinking water, and chlorine is unable to eliminate them.

- The cheapest **bottled water is a very expensive** way to have the amount that is necessary for our daily intake, when compared with even **the most expensive water treatment system**, which will provide higher quality water.

- **Dry skin** is a symptom of dehydration. No matter what kind of skin cream we use it cannot replace the moisture necessary for the skin alone, we also need an adequate amount of water daily.

Golden Principle Number Two

- **Research** in the book by Dr. Joseph M. Price, *Coronaries, Cholesterol, and Chlorine*, states that drinking water which contains **chlorine** can cause **atherosclerosis** which is the main cause of heart disease and stroke.

- **Room temperature** is the healthiest way for the body to receive water. Hot water is destructive to vitamins and minerals in the body and to the water itself. **Very cold water** prevents the absorption of vitamins and minerals. The ideal way to consume water is to have it at the room temperature of the living environment.

- In order to kill **micro organisms** in the water via boiling, it needs to boil for at least 20 minutes and that would give us $1/4$ of the original amount that we started with.

Let me tell you some great news about water that is on its way for all of us. This news has not been published yet and is in its infancy, in spite of the fact that for over ten years scientists from many major countries of the world have been working on it. I am unable to tell you the whole story for two reasons.

- I only heard this via audio information and internet.
- If I tell you the whole story, you would definitely think that ABBAS has gone away with the fairies.

Apparently at this moment in time some scientists have come across a way of purifying water to a degree that was never reached before. This water is called **super-ionised water.** It has 3 extra electrons on the outer orbit of its atomic structure, that's all. Nobody can explain how it works. It came from a group of Turkish Sufi masters. A **Sufi master** is similar to a monk in the Western world and Sufi has its origins in Persia.

Have you ever noticed that when you are interested in something you suddenly see it everywhere? That happened to me, since I was looking for the super-ionised water. About three years ago I received from a friend a little bottle of that water. Half a bottle of it is still in my fridge and it is as clear as crystal. You put a few drops in a litre of water and leave it for 24 hours and it purifies the water. Didn't I tell you that you would not believe me?

There you are, what can I say? I knew you wouldn't believe me. Yet I have seen this water with my own eyes, so I know what I am saying is true, but I cannot explain how that happens. You may be wondering why I am telling you this.

Because, I am imagining, what our world would be like if we had such pure water in our hands? The level of our health would go sky high overnight.

But don't worry, because in the later pages I will share with you a type of water treatment system that is available in Europe, America, Australia and Canada. I am not sure of other countries. If you live in any of the above mentioned countries you can easily purchase it and install it on your drinking water supply.

I wish I could share with you the amount of knowledge I have learned in the past 12 years about water and the importance of good quality water for our health. I have witnessed a significant number of patients who have gained a great deal of wellbeing just by increasing their intake of drinking water daily. Really what I am telling you in these few pages is not even a scratch of the information that is available out there about water, which can improve our health to a greater degree.

Did you know that hot flushes are the symptoms of dehydration?

Did you know that high cholesterol is a symptom of dehydration?

Let me tell you about some of the different systems of water purification. Since there are so many types of water filtering systems, it would take lots of pages to explain about all of them in great detail therefore I am only going to mention the most common ones.

First we can look at **JUG TYPES.**

There are many companies who provide this type of water purification. The system is very simple. It only reduces a small number of organic contaminants, and the filter must be changed frequently.

This system improves, TASTE, ODOUR, and CLARITY, by way of using granulated activated charcoal. The water purification standard that this system provides is called Standard 42, and is not effective if the water has heavy metal or VOCs.

GRANULATED ACTIVATED CARBON

This is a more advanced type of water purification compared to the jug types on the market. There are many companies who supply this kind of water filtration.

Because of the various types available it is not easy to make a reliable statement which can be comprehensive about this system, but one thing is well proven: it does not purify some of the heavy metals, like lead and mercury, and has no effect on inorganic compounds, or harmful micro organisms. Also they do not have '**REVERSE BLOCKED SYSTEMS**'. This means filtered and unfiltered water is in the same container.

WATER SOFTENERS

This system is very effective in terms of the reduction of lime scale in the household use of water. There is added salt, which changes the taste of water but it does not have any effect on any micro organism.

DISTILLATION

This is actually one of the best types of drinking water, if it is not used as the principle daily intake. There are three challenges attached to this system.

It requires enormous amounts of energy to provide a single litre of water.

This purification process removes desirable minerals like calcium and magnesium from the water. Magnesium is needed for balance of electrolytes, which is helpful to regulate body temperature and control blood pressure.

It requires very good discipline to produce the amounts which one needs daily, of water. I have noticed in the past 12 years that people who start to use this system begin with good intentions, then eventually they loose interest and after a while the unit is stored in the garage.

COMPRESSED CARBON BLOCK TECHNOLOGY WITH ULTRAVIOLET LIGHT

This is the most effective one that I have come across, since it has it all in one package. As far as I know this system can remove over 140 possible contaminants from our drinking water. These include lead, mercury, VOCs and the petrol additive MTBE (Methyl Tertiary Butyl Ether). The filter needs to be changed only once a year and satisfies three standards of water purification: Standards 42, 53, and 55.

- Standard 42 includes improvement of TASTE, SMELL, and CLARITY.
- Standard 53 includes the above, plus VOCs and disinfectant by-products.
- Standard 55 includes microbiological water treatment.

As far as I know it is the only water treatment system in the world, which has the ability to perform the above mentioned standards at the point of use from the household tap.

Also this system has been awarded the **GOLD SEAL** by the Water Quality Association, and the NSF which is a not for profit organisation that provides the most comprehensive information about the performance of different water treatment systems in the world.

I think by now you have enough information about water. Again I would like to remind you that any information is only effective when we apply it in our daily life.

Now, let me conclude this chapter. This is all you need to know.

Drink 2 to 3 litres of **PURE, CLEAN, CLEAR, WATER DAILY** and you will soon be healthier. Remember:

WATER IS LIFE!

We Are Always Only One Step Away from Optimal Health

CHAPTER TEN

GOLDEN PRINCIPLE NUMBER THREE

EAT LESS and MOVE MORE

I don't think I need to say more about this, do I? This title says it all. Nevertheless, let's talk about it anyway. But before we get into any technical details, in keeping with the manner of this book so far, let me tell you a story.

The date is approximately 300 BC and somewhere in Greece at that time there lived an outstanding philosopher. I do not know his name in English but he lived at the time of Alexander the Great. He was a very simple man and totally detached from the material world. Alexander the Great was very fond of him.

This philosopher happened to live in a big urn at the edge of a market in a small city. When the sun was out, it shone into the urn and, on rainy days the philosopher would pull the lid over the urn to stop himself from getting wet.

I read this tale in a book of his life almost thirty years ago when I was doing compulsory military service in my country and the story had such an effect on me that I remember it clearly even today.

This strange philosopher did not ask for much in the way of comfort because managing to survive on very little was part of his philosophy. The only thing he possessed apart from his clothes was a cup made of clay that he kept for collecting drinking water from a nearby river or spring. One day, as he went to the spring to fill his cup with water, he noticed a little boy drinking the water out of his hand.

He watched, mesmerised by that simple action, and eventually said: 'People think I am a great philosopher. But today I realise that I am not even as intelligent as this little boy. For all these years I have had something in my possession that I could do without.'

After saying that he threw away the cup and from that day forward his clothes were his only possessions until he died.

Now in comparison to him can you imagine how much we carry around that we could do without? May I suggest that as well as *eating less* we could also try *collecting less*!

I've noticed in the twenty years that I've lived in Western society that we all accumulate so much more than we need. As a result, this affects our general wellbeing. You may well say as you are reading this: 'Come on Abbas! Give us a break! We can't all live like monks!' Well, no, but nobody expects you to live like a monk.

Nonetheless, can you tell me how many of us keep things in our garage or shed that we have no use for anymore. Things that are getting rusty or rotten and yet we still do not give them away? Things like a second kettle or old toasters, etc, etc. Also it is especially true for some of us who have the best intentions to lose weight and so those beautiful jeans that have not fitted for ten years or so, we still keep them in the wardrobe because maybe *someday* they will fit! Do I need to say more? Have you got the picture yet?

Here is a suggestion for you, anyway. Go to your wardrobe or garage and give away anything that you decide is no longer useful. If you find this difficult then perhaps consider another method. Agree that you will help get rid of the things belonging to your husband or wife which are no longer of use and he or she can then do the same for you. You could do this with your children or your parents or friends. Any of them can do it for you. It is especially good to let your children help you with this 'outward' cleaning up.

You're probably thinking: 'What about you, Abbas? How much junk have *you* got that you don't need?'

Who? Me? Well it may surprise you to know that I am the biggest collector of *junk* you can imagine. But my belongings are different. I keep things like a clipping from a health magazine that twenty years ago described the effectiveness of pineapple in preventing heart disease, or how some scientists found that drinking coffee can cause miscarriages, and so on. (*By the way both these statements are absolutely true!*)

Anyway, you would never believe how much paper I manage to keep! I am very glad that computers came along to save me a lot of space, and I now also shred things to use as mulch in the garden.

I am just sharing this with you because we are all culprits of material possessions. They can take us over in effect if we are not careful. Anyway try clearing some of them out and see how you feel about it. Trust me on this! You will not believe until you do it, how great you will feel afterwards. *You see, we are all multi-dimensional beings.* Our surroundings affect our health and wellbeing because they are usually a reflection of what is happening to us on the inside. So quietly ponder these things perhaps for a moment or two before reading on…

And now having done that, let's go back briefly to our story.

Apparently one day Alexander the Great was passing by the philosopher's little city with his army and he stopped to talk to the philosopher. After inspecting the urn and its surroundings, Alexander said: 'I think a great person like you should not live in such humble conditions. I will help you if you like and give you anything you want.'

The philosopher smiled and asked him: 'Will you really promise that?'

Alexander smiled too, his face alight with hope and joy and said: 'Yes, of course I will promise!'

The philosopher nodded gratefully and replied. 'I wonder if you would be kind enough to move over a bit, you and your horse are blocking the sunshine that I was enjoying before you arrived.'

As I said before, the philosopher's life story had an unforgettable effect on me and the reason I wish to share the story with you is because this philosopher also had a famous theory or opinion about food and eating. He is reported to have said once: *'Everybody has portions of food that are allocated to him or her for their entire lifetime.'*

Now that may sound very simple or possibly not make any sense at all. He did explain the idea in great detail over several pages but the essence is as I have spelled it out above. I think there is great wisdom in that opinion and I also feel that most of the allergies we suffer from today may diminish if we apply this idea in our life.

Golden Principle Number Three

When we consume food, our body needs to break it down into small pieces so that it can be absorbed into our bloodstream. From there it can supply nutrients to wherever the body requires them. Now, the way for the body to break down the food into smaller pieces is by chemical reactions. These usually start in our digestive tract via substances called *enzymes* and the definition of an enzyme is; a substance that acts as a catalyst in living organisms, regulating the rate at which chemical reactions proceed without it being altered in the process.

My instinctive belief which I can't prove, is that **humans have been allocated only a certain number of enzymes for their entire life.** Okay, now while keeping that in mind please read the next paragraph.

Also, did you know that **almost all uncooked fruits and vegetables do not need any enzymes to be digested in our body**? The necessary enzymes required in breaking down such fruits or vegetables are already contained within them.

Wellness is exemplified by those who live longest and the Japanese inhabitants of Okinawa are well known for living to an advanced age. This secret of their longevity seems to revolve around that fact that they get up from the table before they are over-full so compared with people in other parts of the world, they 'eat less and move more'.

When we combine these two facts and my own theory about enzymes, perhaps we can start to understand the secrets of longevity. In other words, we can maintain our life energy with foods which *do not* need to use up the enzymes from the deposit account of our body. By consuming smaller amounts of foods requiring enzymes, and larger amounts of those which produce their *own* enzymes, we can possibly live longer by conserving our own amounts of digestive enzymes.

I hope you can follow what I am trying to say because we are now ready to move on to the next category.

When the wise ancient physicians found a new discovery they did not have a scientific way to explain themselves, they used a story to explain their discoveries to others. Since I am unable to either prove or refer to a scientific research about this I am also going to use their way and tell you another story.

Imagine a person lives for a hundred years and the food that is allocated to him or her is as follows: 35,000 apples; 20,000 oranges; 15,000 eggs; 15,000 loaves of bread; 5,000 chickens; 5,000 fish, and so on.

Now you may say what has this got to do with anything? You may recall me mentioning allergies in the beginning of this chapter, so now let me explain allergies and how I understand them. *Firstly*, what is an allergy? The simplest way to describe it is like this. An allergy is actually the body *telling* you: 'I am unable to digest or handle this substance.' Or: 'I've already had too much of it *so please give me a break!*'

Have you ever wondered *why* people who suffer from heart disease are advised to reduce the consumption of fat and rich foods? Could it be possible that they have already eaten too much of these types of foods, and therefore their body is unable to make enzymes to break down those type of foods, this would appear to be the case.

Also another example is a woman who gets recurrent kidney infections has been told to stop drinking coffee? (Just by the way I will mention here that the ill-effects of coffee for women are far greater than for men!) Or why people often have allergy to eggs, or wine, or anything that they frequently enjoy ?

Mostly this happens when they have had a surfeit of something already so there is no reserve of the needed enzyme in their digestive bank. And like our cash flow in the bank, imagine it as a monthly instalment paid into our account from our workplace. What would happen if we spent more than was paid in per month? We'd run out of money, right?

How much better it is to imagine that you only use 80% of your budget every month so that after a few years, you are left with a lot in hand and you can then sustain yourself much longer. I know you may say this sounds so simple. But believe me, it is! If only we could get our head around the idea of *eating less.*

LIVING TO BE ONE HUNDRED – AND HOW TO DO IT!
Here is another way of explaining the subject. Did you know that the only common denominator among centenarians in the world – those people who live to be over 100 years old– is that they eat smaller

portions of food daily compared to others? That's very interesting, isn't it? In other words, by eating smaller amounts, they are expanding their life expectancy! In fact the Japanese people who live in Okinawa *are* the lowest calorie consumers in the entire world.

To date several studies have been carried out to find out why some people live over a hundred years. Some centenarians smoke, some don't, some drink, some don't, some are vegetarian, and some are not, and so on. But the only thing common to them all is that they all eat very little.

There are quite a few cultures in the world where people live to an average of over one hundred years. Amongst them are the Abkhazians, the Azerbaijanis, the Hunzas and, of course the Okinawans. The reason I choose to focus on the Okinawan people from amongst all the other centenarians, is the likely connection between their low calorie diet and the low rate of cancer amongst their women.

Did you know that in Okinawa only six women in every 100,000 suffer from breast cancer? This is very small in comparison to the Western world where the rate is one in seven. That is a rather frightening statistic, isn't it?

Now we are beginning to know much more about the value and importance of a stress-free lifestyle and are learning also how to protect ourselves against disease via the use of supplements. So there are many other factors that can contribute towards our longevity that we can take advantage of to support us in our daily lives. You can easily find much of the above information on the Internet or from your local library.

By now I think you should have a good idea of the advantages that can accrue to you by **EATING LESS** – and the powerful benefits that one can get from this philosophy. If you are still not convinced, then you will find out more when reading the following chapter on Nutrition.

Please remember we only retain a small percentage of our total daily food consumption, and we even lose that small amount within 60 to 120 days from our total body weight which becomes new cells because we release it in the form of dead cells and carbon dioxide. However, that is the good news. Can you imagine what size we would be if we retained more than that?

Now let me say that if you are still not totally convinced about the *power of eating less*, then I would like to share with you this trick that I heard about at a motivational talk which I attended some years ago. It goes something like this: From tomorrow whenever you desire a big meal or a nice slice of cake or some other delicious looking food that has been put in front of you, please sit down in front *of* a mirror and eat it without any clothes on ! I should perhaps add that I have not tried this myself yet. If you do, perhaps you will let me know how effective it was for you!

THE LOGIC OF SENSIBLE EATING

I think it may help here to talk for a moment about food in a more logical way. There are so many books written about food, diet, recipes, and so on that it is difficult to be totally definitive. Nevertheless I would like to share with you my own understandings that have been gained over quite a few years of dealing with clients and their health challenges.

It seems obvious that we consume food for two reasons. Firstly we eat for energy and nourishment and secondly for enjoyment. At least I can see no other reasons except these two. Now let me analyse my experience and I hope it will be interesting for you.

We consume meat, potatoes, fruits and vegetables in order to get protein, carbohydrate, vitamins, minerals and fibre. Indeed, during the process of consuming food hopefully we are enjoying it, and that is great. But the enjoyment cannot be the most important part, it must be secondary. If we only focus on the enjoyment of eating in itself, then we are going to end up with illnesses.

We eat chocolate. *Why?* Because we enjoy it! But our bodies do not need confectionary chocolate, right? That is why we end up with all kinds of allergic reactions to it. Another example of this problem is that people like to consume alcohol, particularly in Western society. Its consumption is purely for enjoyment and socialising and often I am asked by my clients: 'Will it be all right to have it in moderation?'

Now moderation is a tricky word, since it can be adjusted to suit any of our wrong eating habits, or any other activities which we carry out. In fact I have noticed that the issue of moderation is usually raised by

Golden Principle Number Three

people when what they really wish to say is: 'Can I continue doing what I am doing and still be okay?'

Well, at the end of the day it is our body. We may be able to fool others but we can never fool ourselves. Most of us, deep down, know what is good for our health and what is not, but still continue to eat the wrong foods. If we do eat the wrong foods, maybe the question we need to ask ourselves is this: 'Why do I find it difficult to control myself when it comes to what I put into my body? I am sure there are many examples you can think of where it is not the lack of knowledge, but will power that is the missing piece.

Commercial advertising works by promising us pleasures that we can gain from certain products and unfortunately most of us fall for these adverts! Nonetheless, there are no products advertised that I know of that are so harmful that it would concern me too much. What does concern me more is our attitude towards eating them in general.

One attitude, which particularly concerns me, is seeing the digestive tract simply as a pipe that starts from our mouth and ends up in our anus. We sometimes seem to think that we are here in this life for the express purpose of eating our way through all the foods of the world via that pipe. As a result of all this eating from time to time the pipe becomes blocked. Then we make every effort to open the pipe so as to *keep on* eating. Then we become ill, so we go for some medicine.

I think you will have got the point now from this little tirade of mine. And I hope it wasn't too graphic for you! Yet this sort of attitude is fairly widespread and possibly one of the reasons why our hospitals are always overflowing with sick and unwell people. So I want to pause to summarise a little here. The key point of this chapter of course is to encourage you to *eat less and move more.* To help with the 'eating less' aspect of this vital maxim I am going to spell out what are perhaps the six most important areas for attention.

THE SIX FIRST SUBSTANCES TO REDUCE
You can start by reducing just six substances in your regular diet, which will quickly help you to gain a great deal of wellness. Those six substances are: **TEA, COFFEE, ALCOHOL, CIGARETTES, SUGAR**

and SALT. I shall give a short explanation of each of the substances and talk about the link between them and some pathologies or illnesses. Please at least try to cut them down to a half or a quarter of your present use. Also I suggest that next time you go to your doctor, ask him or her if you need to be concerned about malnutrition when reducing the six above-mentioned substances. I can assure you that he or she will agree with me that this is a good suggestion. Let's look at them in turn.

ALCOHOL

Did you know that we also produce dopamine in our bodies when we consume alcohol? But the feel good factor only lasts for 20 minutes. After that all we have is a light headache – and no matter how much more alcohol we drink, the feeling is the same. I know I am entering a very sensitive area, but I have to speak the truth of my heart.

Please remember I am not saying it is *right* or *wrong* to drink alcohol. I am simply looking at it objectively. The many side effects of alcohol cannot be denied, particularly the ill effects it can have on family life, communication, and on children, when parents consume large amounts.

I cannot personally find any good in the consumption of alcohol, despite the fact that a large amount of our wealth is being spent on it. Most people excuse it as a means of socialising. But whilst every culture in the world needs to socialise not all of them use alcohol.

Another excuse is that it is okay if consumed in 'moderation'. Now hold on there for a moment, I find I can tolerate moderation for everything else but have a challenge when it comes to alcohol and I will tell you why. When we eat any food we eventually feel full, but when we consume alcohol we tend to lose control of the amount that we can drink. I know there are some exceptions and certain people seem to have greater control than others – especially those who suffer from the after-effects. But generally speaking, we do not have a great control over alcohol.

You see when we consume alcohol, after only a few minutes the molecules of alcohol enter our blood via our stomachs and although the thick blood vessel walls can protect our brains from most toxins

Golden Principle Number Three

entering our bloodstream, alcohol particles are so small that within seconds they enter into our brain and cut off the neurotransmissions between cells. Therefore, after a few minutes, we lose control of our higher brain and are left with only our animal brain. And after we drink an amount equal to fourteen glasses of beer, we lose control of our animal brain too.

I know some friends who have a great way of preventing themselves from drinking too much. They take only small amounts of money with them when they go out for a drink! This is a very good trick but would you be able to refuse if someone with whom you are enjoying a conversation offers to pay for your drink?

If your answer is: 'Yes, I can control myself', then congratulations! You are rare and a very strong person, since in my experience only a few people can control themselves in such circumstances. Well let's get the point clear, and see what we can do so as to have our joy without paying such a heavy price afterwards.

Where alcohol is concerned it is more important than ever to remember the title of this chapter which is the Third Golden Principle of Wellness: **EAT LESS & MOVE MORE!** That in essence is all we need to remember. The rest is up to you; find yourself a way that suits your personality and lifestyle. In short I will say to anybody who drinks alcohol, please do your best to reduce your weekly intake by a half or a quarter of your present use. This way you will save money and have the possibility of having a longer, more joyful and hopefully healthier life, too.

There are different levels of addiction to alcohol and there is one very interesting feature that I have found is common to all levels: **that when we are really addicted, we believe we can stop at any time.** That belief usually goes hand in hand with another twin belief: that we never actually feel that we are addicted to the particular substance in the first place. That is why many keep on going until one day we realise with a **BANG** that we have an addiction, and of course it is too late.

I recently heard an amusing statement by a man who was being interviewed on Irish National Radio on the subject of addictions. The substance being discussed was hashish and the man in question made this statement, 'I have been smoking hashish for over twenty-five years and I am not addicted to it' this was said in all seriousness and I will leave you to absorb the subtle humour of that statement.

I will sometime perhaps write about my clinical observations of people I have treated for various addictions as in most cases the results have been very encouraging. However that is maybe for another time, possibly another book. Meantime let's turn to the next important substance that we can reduce.

TEA

It is important to reduce tea in our daily diet – particularly if we suffer from any of the following pathologies: *PMS* or *PMT*– premenstrual syndrome or premenstrual tension being more or less the same thing – all kinds of *arthritis, backache, headaches and multiple sclerosis.*

If you suffer from any of these illnesses you definitely need to reduce your daily intake of tea. Please let me make it clear that I am not suggesting that drinking tea is the cause of these symptoms, but it certainly does not help them. As I have already mentioned above, so that you may have confidence in what I am saying, please check with your doctor about the value of cutting down on the six substances I refer to here. In my experience most doctors are very reasonable and understanding – and it is in their interest also of course that you should get well!

COFFEE

The amount of coffee that is currently consumed in Western society is more than TOO MUCH! However, for some African and South American countries, a high percentage of their exports to the Western world are tea and coffee. Their economies are so dependent on these products that one has to be careful how to talk about this subject without upsetting the economic and trade apple cart, so to speak. Anyway, I'll share with you some of my clinical observations and research and leave any judgment up to you.

I was listening to a domestic radio programme at home, (which between intervals of music gives brief reports on various scientific research projects). One day I heard a mention of a report that said that

Golden Principle Number Three

drinking coffee can reduce heart attacks. So I checked up on their research protocol and found that in fact several bad effects from drinking coffee had also been listed, yet the radio programme or the researchers had chosen to only mention the one finding, in favour of drinking coffee, for some reason.

When in Africa working on a project concerning solar-dried fruits and vegetables we were all sitting around during our midday break drinking water, eating fresh fruit and chewing on kola nuts or coffee beans. I hardly ever saw anyone drinking instant coffee while I was there and maybe this was due to the heat. The way coffee was used amongst the Bushmen I worked with, was to have two or three beans only, to chew on.

In our modern, Western lifestyle, of course, the way we consume coffee is so different, and the amount we use is so much greater – dangerously so, in my opinion. People often drink coffee to get energised since of course it gives a quick and artificial 'high'. So much so that, after a few years of drinking it regularly, it easily becomes an addiction and it is not unusual under these circumstances for people to be unable to function properly in the morning, unless they have had a few cups of coffee.

Here for your reference are some key points on the negative effects caused by drinking too much coffee:

- Depletes vitamins and minerals from our body.
- Interferes with our stomach juices and makes the digestion tract weaker.
- Artificially stimulates adrenalin, and weakens our kidneys and our urinary tract.
- Depletes the substance which lubricates our joints, called synovial fluid, by crystallizing it. As a result, people who drink a lot of coffee may find that they suffer pain in their joints and a cracking noise on movement.
- Coffee contains a substance called caffeine or cafestol. This substance accelerates the production of chemicals in our body called free radicals, in other words, aging chemicals. The funny thing is that decaffeinated coffee has more cafestol than ordinary coffee.

My wife Carmel and I occasionally love to have a cappuccino. But we drink just four or five cups a year – that's right only that much in a whole year! It might be when we go on a trip or for some special occasion. Then we drink it and we really enjoy it. I am not suggesting you have to do the same as we do but you might find something else that suits you. Reducing the amount of coffee you drink can only benefit your health.

Now here are some suggestions for those people who would otherwise find it difficult to reduce their coffee intake:

- Try making a half-cup of coffee, but four times stronger than you normally make it and with no milk or sugar. Allow it to cool, then using a teaspoon take a drop every few minutes. Do this four or five times, you will get the same 'kick' from the caffeine, but without so much of the ill effects.
- You could also try a coffee substitute called Guarana, since it will give the same or even better energy than coffee. It increases the efficiency of the circulation rather than artificially stimulating adrenalin. I am sure you can find it at most Health Food stores.
- There is also an herbal tea called MATE that is another source of caffeine but not as strong as commercial instant coffee.
- Another technique is to place five or six cardamom pods in your coffee and chew them after you have finished drinking it. This offers some antidote to the ill-effects of the caffeine.

SMOKING

I feel there is more than enough bad news about smoking to make any smoker depressed. Often, the bad news can have a negative effect on the smoker because it takes away any enjoyment and peace of mind that smoking can bring! So, in this section I will tell you all the information, you may see as *good* news that I know about smoking.

The first, 'good news' – for smokers and maybe even the tobacco companies – is that scientists in Europe have discovered a vaccine which can block the harmful chemical, nicotine, from going to the brain. Currently it is on trial and it is hoped that soon they can eliminate the harmful effects of smoking.

On a personal note, I remember one summer evening my wife and I were staying at a hotel in Dublin. When I opened a window, I saw a man sitting outside on his own smoking a cigarette. He had a beer on the table in front of him and I couldn't help watching him as once every few seconds, he would inhale the cigarette smoke, totally lost in the joy of smoking. It was almost as if he was meditating. I thought the cruellest thing would be to tell him that smoking causes cancer and possibly ruin his joy. I asked my wife to come and look at how the man was enjoying his smoking. Eventually I said to her, 'Would you believe it, this scene made me feel like I would take up smoking again if I thought there were no harmful side-effects!'

I had in mind of course everything from the unpleasant smell smoking causes on an individual's breath and clothes, in work places and homes, to the high risk of cancer that comes from smoking, also the negative effect it has on passive smokers. Unfortunately these are inescapable facts.

Another good thing that may be said about smoking is that it is not truly an addiction, it is a habit. Most smokers have a pattern when they have a cigarette. For example, to smoke after a nice meal is a strong desire of most smokers. Imagine that after dinner you sit down on the couch, open a packet of cigarettes, light up – with a lighter which gives a much nicer feeling than with matches, I think, and you have your cup of tea or coffee beside you, and maybe you decide to turn on the television as well. Or maybe you chose to listen to some soft music and ... I can go on giving a description of the whole night for you if you wish!

What I've just described of course is called a smoker's comfort zone and it is this which we find challenging to give up. The pattern, the process, the ritual – all of this makes up the habit. This is why it is so difficult to give up and why *so* many people go back to cigarettes after they quit. Cigarettes are the main players in the ritual, so trying to do without them is like trying to cook a meal without heat.

In spite of the thousands of books written on how to give up smoking, very few can offer a way to fill the vacuums left in our daily routines when we do. As I hinted before, sometime I will write a comprehensive book about addictions in general and smoking in particular and I will set down all my clinical observations and the way I approach these issues. But for now here are some brief suggestions on how to deal with reducing smoking while we are reducing all these other substances in our diet in this section.

It is necessary to start by thinking of **breaking the habit.**

In order to do this, you need to be constantly changing your habits. For example, if you love smoking after a meal, you need to do something else first after the meal– then smoke. Let's say that every time you eat lunch or dinner you light a cigarette straight afterwards. What you need to do is to break that habit. You might try going for a walk first or washing the dishes or cleaning the kitchen or anything else that needs doing. Whatever it is, do that *first* before you sit down and smoke. Choose different things each time to avoid doing the same actions twice in a row.

Another technique that I find extremely helpful in many cases is this: decide on the number of cigarettes you smoke daily no matter how many it is. Let's say you like to smoke twenty a day. Just decide on that number and stick to it. Then next decide on a time limit. Now tell yourself that for three months, say, you are going to smoke that number and *no more.* Then try to stay with that amount, *no matter what happens* – even if you are at a wedding and you finish your twenty cigarettes by five p.m.! When you have finished your daily quota, do whatever you can to occupy yourself so that you *do not break* the agreement on the number.

The other side of the coin is that you should not break that agreement even if you have smoked *less* than your chosen number by the end of the day. For example, maybe you are ready to go to bed and you have only smoked fifteen cigarettes that day out of your agreement of twenty. What you *then* need to do is smoke the remainder so that you still keep to your agreed number per day.

Golden Principle Number Three

It is very important for you to follow the instructions *exactly* as described above. The theory behind this perhaps calls for a deeper explanation but since there is not enough time and space here at this point in this book, I shall give you a simplified version of it which I will call:

BEING IN THE DRIVER'S SEAT.
Imagine you are on a bus, and the driver brings the bus along his allocated route. You have no choice because you are a passenger and have no control over the speed or the destination. The only choice you have is to get off the bus, but that is not what you want to do since outside is wet and cold and there is no other bus around, and so you stay on.

In this story the bus is, of course, symbolic of the smoking routine that you are familiar with, either at home or in your social environment. You seem to have no control over it, which is why you smoke a certain number, and when your environment changes your smoking pattern changes with it.

For example, if you are taking a long flight and there is a *No Smoking* policy on the plane, you have no choice for many hours but to avoid smoking. On the other hand, when you are with a friend at a wedding, or you are socialising, you may find you smoke *more* than you usually do.

You see, you are not in the driver's seat and what actually dictates your smoking is your environment. By choosing a certain number of cigarettes to smoke and keeping to it you go in the driver's seat: in other words, you are at the controls.

I have found that the hardest part of the process of giving up smoking for most people is breaking the habit, the routine, and the rituals. In fact, based on testimonies of many cases that I have worked with, it appears that the giving up or reducing of smoking is easier than to change one's cherished regime.

You need to know that, when you stick to your chosen number of cigarettes, your higher brain takes over from your animal brain and, before you know, one day you can stop smoking with very little or no effort at all. Finally, the most important thing to remember is: to let *go* of any guilty feelings you may have when you smoke. You see, it is not only the smoking which can kill you! But your attitude to smoking and feeling guilty about it plays a big part also.

Now perhaps this is a good point at which to tell another story before I conclude this section on smoking by summarising my three main suggestions for dealing with the problem of reducing it. This particular tale is called:

THE STORY OF SHAH ABBAS

One day Shah Abbas, one of the great past kings of Persia, posed this question to two men, Sheikh Baha'i and Mirdamad, who was the brother-in-law of the shah or king.

'Which of the following three things has more value: the teaching of manners and education, the power of basic instincts or the power of noble birth and integrity?'

Sheikh Baha'i answered without hesitation, 'In my view, it is unquestionably the power of basic instinct.'

But when Mirdamad answered he insisted otherwise, 'No, I feel certain it is the power of teaching manners and education.'

So the Shah decided that the Sheikh and Mirdamad should carry out an experiment to see which answer was the correct one. Each made their separate preparations and the day came when they were ready to test their experiment in front of the shah.

Mirdamad had ordered a trained cat to be brought in, one who had not eaten for hours. He placed some food in front of the cat and commanded her not to eat. Where upon the cat obeyed the order and did not move. The Shah was very pleased and quite surprised by the power and success of Mirdamad's training and education.

Next it was the turn of the Sheikh to respond to the experiment and he bowed to the Shah before asking servants to bring in the same cat and feed her. This they did until the cat was unable to eat any more. Then the Sheikh released, onto the floor of the palace, a mouse which he had hidden in his pocket. The frightened little mouse ran as fast as she could to escape but the cat chased after the mouse.

So Sheikh Baha'I' asked Mirdamad, 'Will you please order the cat to stop.'

Mirdamad loudly ordered the trained cat to stop – but this time there was no way the cat would do as it was told. It was as if the cat had suddenly grown deaf and chased the mouse as its ancestors had done since time immemorial!

You can perhaps see how this story can lead to many interesting discussions on how the minds of men and animals operate. At first, the shah had been delighted by the obedience of the cat. It seemed to him that if a *cat* could be trained thus, so could many of his subjects. But when the cat did not obey the second command, he grew confused.

I have told this story because I would like to share with you, through it, some of my understanding of the human mind and its complexities. You see, nowadays prisons are full of people who did not manage to control their basic human or animal instincts. At the instant their crime was committed, it seems their animal brain took over and they lost control, although this is not perhaps true invariably in all cases.

In fact, people who commit a crime seldom have a pleasant memory of the incident. If they do, that in itself is considered an illness. More usually they regret what they have done, and the misery they inflict on themselves by their action can be even worse than the misery inflicted on others.

There are innumerable theories as to why some of us behave in such a way, and very few satisfactory answers present themselves. Often, the idea is that if we recognise the problem we can find a solution. But unfortunately this does not appear to be true in most cases, as in our story.

The cat certainly wasn't chasing the mouse for food or to satisfy her hunger. There was an even more basic instinct at work in her and this is described well in ancient Persian writings I am very fond of, which say: Those hidden undesirable forces are like black ants which are asleep on a black stone in a dark night. Let us pray that they will never waken.

I would like to share with you the way that I myself, most of the time, succeed in controlling those hidden undesirable forces and that is by prayer and meditation. This works for me and it is the only solution I know. I cannot be sure it would work for everybody, but for me it is simple and effective. It certainly will do no harm to try it yourself.

I am sure people know of other techniques which they may use to overcome their weakness in moments of crisis, and I would love to hear your own ideas. But please excuse me, I have digressed a little from our original discussion about smoking, habits and addictions, so now let's return to out main theme.

If you are a smoker I would ask you to look at why you chose to smoke. Is it because your friends did? Does it make you feel relaxed? Do you feel okay with putting a harmful substance into your body? Or do you feel bad about it?

I believe that how one feels about smoking also has an effect on our health alongside the harmful substance itself. So here is a summary of my suggestions for those who smoke which I believe will help reduce the harmful effects, help you to stop smoking if you choose to, and to take the control back.

- When you do smoke, enjoy it and avoid guilty feelings.
- Chose a suitable number of cigarettes per day and stay with it – indefinitely.
- Break the habit by constantly changing your personal smoking routine.

And above all, don't worry since worry brings about fear and fear is crippling. Please remember that nothing is bad in itself. It is only in our minds that we interpret something as good or bad. We do the same through our beliefs, which are given to us by our parents or our culture or from scientific research. An example of how received wisdom can change is the early medical practice of lancing or blood-letting. Once it was the science of its day; now it is considered barbaric behaviour. Furthermore modern scientific research also has a similar habit of changing its view point, sometimes within a few years, and often forgets to tell the public when it has contradicted itself.

Anyway I trust I am explaining myself to you. In any event it is important always to remember that control over your health is first and foremost in your own hands. And in general terms we are always **only one step away from optimal health.**

Now let's move on from the disadvantages of smoking to the disadvantages associated with **sugar.**

SUGAR

When I use the term 'sugar' I mean any kind of sweetener, sweets of all kinds and any other sugary things. Traditionally sweets are a way of expressing love for others, particularly when given by the elderly to small children. Most people have childhood memories of their Granny or Grandpa giving them sweets. In this connection I feel it is worth saying: **'It is not too late to have a happy childhood!'**

I interpret this as meaning that you have a choice over the memories you bring with you from childhood. You can choose or decide to bring with you the *best* memories and 'play' them over and over until they are a part of you. It took me years to understand the value of this and though you may view it differently, this sentence helped me greatly to recognise the best things in my own childhood.

One of those great – and *sweet* – memories from childhood that has always remained with me is of my own Granny. What a remarkable and wise person she was! One day my Grandpa went out travelling somewhere and was going to be staying away for a few days. I of course, being a small child, wanted to go with him. When he replied 'No, you can't' this upset me greatly and I began to cry. We were at the bus station and Granny gently asked me to stop crying and said that she would buy something nice for me later. Of *course,* the bribe worked! I believe I was around five or six years old at the time.

After we had said our goodbyes to my Grandpa, she brought me to the market. There she purchased for me some golden seedless grapes of excellent quality and one expensive yellow pear that in everyday life we could not usually afford. Believe me when I tell you how I still remember the taste of that fruit, even though it is now more than forty years ago. Her wise action created such a strong memory in me that, when I now treat myself, I always buy some lovely fruit as this makes me feel good.

Do notice how parents today tend to buy treats for their children that are not normally considered good for them. These are often sweets, chocolate, crisps and so on – such things that the child has already learned are bad for their teeth and their general wellbeing. So what sort of a subliminal message is that to the child?

Maybe this is why, when we grow up, we consume all kinds of food and drink that we know can harm us, but to which we still find it difficult to say: 'No'. When we say: 'I am going to treat myself', we usually go out and look for something that is harmful to our health! I should give a mention here of some women who are wise in the way they treat themselves, and buy diamonds or nice clothes or a weekend away.

Now, having got all that off my chest, let's talk about the effects that sweets can have on our body. In Ancient Persia and Greece, treatment for the body was always begun with food. And foods were generally separated into four groups as follows: **SWEET, SOUR, BITTER** and **SALTY.**

The physician, in those days, would try to find a link between one of the four types of food eaten and the symptoms revealed at the time of diagnosis. He then gave advice on that basis. The colour of a person's skin could also be a key to analysing the condition of the gallbladder. The amount of bile secreted by the gallbladder was very significant to the treatment. I mention this here, to emphasise the interdependence of the four food types and the importance of consuming them in the right proportions.

In my past twenty years of working, studying and observing the diet of different nations, I have noticed that people in the West consume a large amount of sweet and salt foods, very little sour and hardly any bitter foods at all. Significantly, a large proportion of the population of Europe and America suffers from endless allergic reactions and a variety of illnesses. The ancient doctors I am referring to would say that what

Golden Principle Number Three

we must do to eliminate such problems, is to maintain the correct balance between all the four food types mentioned above.

As to the appropriate quantities for each individual, this will depend upon differences of age and environment, or any predisposition to disease, usually referred to as hereditary factors. All such factors need to be carefully considered before advice for the appropriate quantity can be given. Nevertheless, what is important to understand here is that sweets of all kinds are detrimental to our health when we consume too much of them.

You may well ask how much the right amount to consume is. Well, if we are referring to the white, refined, processed product or *everyday* sugar, the answer is none at all. But how can we realistically handle this when faced with all the temptations and abundance of so much sweet stuff on the market, not to mention the endless problem of *added sugar* in all our processed and packaged food.

I have already noticed that trying to cut it out of our diet altogether does not usually work. Instead, I suggest cutting back or reducing one's intake to a half or even a quarter of the amount that you currently use. In this connection I wish to make a very heartfelt plea to you which will possibly surprise and delight you a little, **please, please, please never give up sweets altogether!**

You should know that sweet things are 'the answer' to our only real vulnerability among the four food types. They can actually fill an emotional and mental vacuum in us. Since we have so little control over our need for sweet things, I suggest it is as well to continue eating them just a little and I really mean a very small amount...

In fact it is worth saying this: Most people have a SWEET TOOTH! Indeed, the human preference for sweets is thought to be a basic survival adaptation. When presented with a variety of basic tastes such as sweet, salty, bitter or sour, infants favour the sweet choice. Scientists believe this preference may be an evolutionary design that ensures infants accept life-sustaining milk with its slightly sweet taste that comes from milk sugar or lactose.

121

Excuse Me! Is This Your Body?

We do need to know, however, that a small amount, whilst not harmful in itself, may give rise to avoidable consequences later on. Let me illustrate this with a simple example. Have you ever tried to hold your finger under a tap which is leaking? Did you notice the pressure when you tried to stop it? The amount of water leaking is so small, and yet it soon becomes impossible to stop so that, after a few seconds of holding it, the water pressure will finally push your finger away.

This is worth remembering about the consumption of sweet things in our daily life. Do it, but only in small amounts! In fact make it almost nothing in comparison to what is presently consumed, and when I say small amounts I really mean it! The consumption of sugar is so high in the Western diet that a quarter of what is now consumed is more than plenty. I remember in 1990, there was a survey in Ireland on the consumption of sugar per person, per year. The results were frightening, particularly in the county of Kilkenny where I live. There the consumption of sugar was one hundred and twenty kg per person, per year!

Now does it make sense to you when I say we consume too much sugar? As a result of which, we have all the illnesses associated with this food type...

Did you know that if you injected the same amount of diluted refined sugar that you consume each day directly into your blood stream, you would still have tooth decay? This is because sugar in all its forms in large amounts depletes calcium from the body. The bones lose their structure and cannot function properly anymore. Maybe that is why humans are the only species with false teeth.

Be that as it may, now that you have been made aware of all the dangers to health from over-consumption of sugary things, I'll try to offer you some sensible alternatives:

- If possible, use honey instead of white sugar.
- Use figs, dates and other dried fruits on a regular basis.
- If you desire sweet things all the time, then you should drink liquorice tea, since a strong desire for sweets points to the inability of

the pancreas to break down sugar. Liquorice tea contains a substance called chromium that activates the pancreas so your blood sugar stays in balance. This in turn reduces the craving for sweets.

- When you eat sweet things, try to have a long walk or do some active work at least within the next two to four hours after eating. This will allow your body to make immediate use of the sugar, preventing it from turning into carbohydrate or partitioning fat.
- If you have a sweet tooth, try to increase your daily consumption of fresh fruit, particularly grapes as they have one of the most balanced sugar contents I know. Half a kilo a day is enough.
- Don't try to give up sweets completely. If you eat just a few you won't feel in denial, but neither will you be damaging your health in the long term

SALT

This is one of the most controversial substances that I have come across in all my years of working in healthcare. Often my clients ask me: 'Is salt good or bad?'

I wish I could find the answer as easily as the question arises. One day we read about how salt is a most essential substance in our diet. Then a few months later we read of its unbelievable harm! It took me years to realise that the problem lies with understanding this substance. Finally I found a way to know the correct amount of salt to use and to advise others appropriately.

I remember in Persia, I used to take one teaspoon of *seawater*, three times a day, as suggested by an Old Persian traditional healer. I do the same today but now I use filtered seawater that has passed through a 'carbon block' filter which has added sea salt because I now know why he suggested that method. Here is the reason:

To truly understand the function of salt, we need to look to the sea; witness the high level of health of its creatures and compare its composition to that of human body fluids. Dead Sea clay contains over eighty elements and most of them are required for the maintenance of the human body.

My interpretation of this is: if Dead Sea clay has over eighty elements in it, then seawater itself must have them in a much more easily assimilated form for human consumption.

We should also remember the cycle through which water travels. It starts by evaporating from the sea to the clouds; then it changes to rain and falls back to the land and into the sea. And on its way back into the sea, it washes everything along with it, including the minerals and trace elements from the land. Since it empties all this into the sea, seawater itself must be a very rich source of minerals. I often wonder what Christ meant when he said to his disciples:

Ye are the salt of the earth: but if the salt has lost its savour, wherewith shall it be salted?
King James Bible, Matthew 5:13

Salt is good: but if the salt has lost its savour, wherewith shall it be seasoned?
King James Bible, Luke 14:34

I wonder if Jesus meant that salts are the preservers of the earth. Or could he also have meant that salt is good if it is in its most complete state? Would it also be right to say that salt preserves the health of our body and the lack of it might be the cause of all kinds of illnesses, a sign, moreover, that the body is beginning to decompose?

You see, salt has a unique structure which is unmistakable. It carries two opposite sides within it, like a hard side and a soft side. Imagine a rock hard wall made from salt, impossible to pass through. But run some water on it and that wall will melt away and eventually become totally dissolved by the water.

Have you ever noticed that some people have minds similar to this? They can appear so strong in their outer expression but, as soon as some emotional crisis occurs in their lives, they totally lose their identity and surprise others with their behaviour.

In homeopathy this is known as the law of signature.

In other words, there is a sign for everything. If we look, observe and

Golden Principle Number Three

study, then it will become obvious to us. In homoeopathy we use this technique a lot to get to the root of the patient's problem, that which is causing him pain and suffering.

Here, then, is my attitude to salt:

Salt is not good or bad; we just need to know how to use it.

I know you are going to say: 'Dah! And shrug just like my two daughters do when they hear an obvious statement. Yet if you eat meat two or three times a week – by that I mean any form of animal meat, fish, chicken, red meat, or especially pork – you do not need to add any salt to your food because you already have enough in your diet.

If, however, you are a vegetarian, you need to add some salt to your diet. Please remember that the only type of salt that is relatively good for human consumption is **SEA SALT**. Sometimes I advise my clients to add almost half a teaspoon of salt to their daily diet, and at other times I ask them to give up using salt altogether. Perhaps this may sound confusing! However it is true to say that we do need to use it correctly since medicine for one person can become poison for another.

I learned this by seeing a lot of National Geographic programmes, which showed elephants, deer and other herbivores travelling for days in order to find salt, though their predators did not seek it at all. This made me think, 'Are we any different from those animals in our need for salt?'

I also noticed that my clients who were not vegetarian did not need to add salt to their diet. If they did, they tended to have problems caused by an excess of salt. However, my vegetarian clients tended to experience the symptoms normally associated with a lack of salt: easily tired; skin breaking out in pimples; and easily catching colds and flu.

If you are in any of the above categories, you need to reconsider your salt intake. Let me just pause for a moment to give you some examples to clarify my point.

Let us say if you are vegetarian and working as a traffic police officer in a hot country you will need a teaspoon of sea salt in your daily diet. If not, you will possibly, as indicated above, suffer skin pimples, constant tiredness and catch cold and flu easily. On the other hand, if you eat meat or have a full Irish or English breakfast even once a week, you do not need salt at all because you already have in your diet more than your body needs. These are relatively easy things to understand. But in other cases it is not so cut and dried.

For a person who does not use salt at all and eats very little meat but has arteriosclerosis (hardening of the arteries), salt is the main cause of his or her problems. In fact, this is one of the most complicated issues connected with salt. According to the medical books there are no real ways of curing this problem through drugs. Yet this problem can be prevented, or in some cases reversed, by the daily consumption of pure, clean, clear water – a quantity of say, two to three litres a day. It is important to know that even a small amount of salt in the human system without **enough water** can cause problems as it will form into a paste.

Here is an example of a lady over fifty years of age who whilst going through the so-called 'change of life' and suffering from hot flushes, has cramps in her lower legs, and feels restless at night. She needs to reduce her salt intake to zero, or increase her intake of water to as much as two to three litres a day.

The whole subject of salt in the diet is one of the most debated topics in the scientific community. Put quite simply, too much salt will undermine our cells metabolism, as will an insufficiency of water. To overcome these problems, if there is very little salt in our body we either can add sea salt to our diet or add some form of sea vegetable like kombu, wakame, hijiki deilisk, kelp, carrageen or any others depending on their availability. Please also note that by eating one head of celery a week the ratio of sodium to potassium in the body stays in the correct balance. This prevents the problem of having too much or too little salt in the body.

If you are a person who needs salt, it is much better I believe to add it to food while it is being cooked, try to avoid shaking salt on your food. The reason for this is when salt is in water or heated it will dissolve into smaller and more digestible particles, particularly if you put salt in water and leave it at least 20 minutes plus. Then it is easier for the body to use it. But when you shake it on to your food, it then becomes difficult for the body to break it down. When salt is used more than the body has need for, or when there is not enough of it, either way can cause all kinds of health problems. If you wish to know more about salt and its use in the body I will highly recommend Dr. B's book (**Water & Salt Your Healers from Within**).

To clarify further the importance of understanding salt and its function, I will share with you my learning of it...

The problem with salt is not the salt itself, but the condition of the salt. In the 1940s the major salt producers in the USA began to dry salt at very high temperatures. This changed the chemical structure of the salt. These changes affect the human body adversely. In order to make salt whiter, dryer and easier to pour they removed the minerals and other nutrients so that what was left was pure white sodium. Sodium is only one chemical found in salt but it is what we buy in our supermarkets and what we erroneously call salt.

Modern scientists have studied the effect of sodium and salt on the human body. It is now widely known that certain substances increase our appetite. Salt is one of the most powerful. The reason for this lies in the part of our brain called the appestat. The appestat constantly monitors the nutrient content of our blood and only when 51 specific nutrients are present at their proper levels will we feel full. Food scientists have found that by adding or subtracting some of these nutrients, they can manipulate our sense of hunger and satiety. While some of this research is still incomplete, it is believed that adding excess fat, sugar and salt to a food tends to make people overeat. To simplify, if we eat a partial food or in the case of salt, a chemical, our brains tell us to keep eating until the correct number of nutrients are present in the blood. Have you ever wondered why you can't eat just one potato chip?

This may help in understanding from another angle what I have said before: that salt is one of the most controversial substances that I have come across in all my years of practice. So here are my final suggestions and conclusions for the time being about salt.

- If you have a habit of putting salt on your food look at what is on your plate. If you are about to eat meat you do not need salt. If you are a person who needs salt, as suggested above, add it to your cooking. That would be one way of helping you to overcome the habit of adding salt freshly to your foods.
- If you need salt then add it when cooking or put a quarter teaspoon into your water jug, for each litre.
- Try to only use sea salt.
- If you are not vegetarian and insist on adding salt to your food, then you need to increase your daily water intake.

Finally one last reminder about the truly vital importance of the title of this chapter, the whole crux of the Third Golden Principle of Wellness and Good Health, '**Eat less and Move More**'. And that would be the key elements for us to remember and try to apply it for the six above mentioned substances.

MOVE MORE

I have quite deliberately chosen to keep these two injunctions tied closely together as one general principle and I wish here to explain that more fully. Firstly, let's talk about the move more part. If you already participate in sporting activities or you regularly exercise at least two or three times a week, then there is not much to be concerned about in relation to your activity levels. What you are doing is probably good enough. But for the rest of us, we need to learn to get our act together regarding the 'move more' part, if we really wish to have a healthy lifestyle.

A good way to start is to walk after food for at least ten to twenty minutes. If possible, go for a walk first thing in the morning or last thing at night before going to bed, whichever suits you best. Or even do both. But make an effort to do it regularly, and keep to the same amount of time each day. Nothing is as powerful as consistency, and after a while it will become second nature. Since we are creatures of habit, it is as well to create some good habits!

If you live in the countryside, then you have no excuse for not going for a walk. Try to look around and enjoy your surroundings. Notice the birds and the trees.

If you choose to go for a walk with a friend or partner, try to focus your conversations on your surroundings, rather than talking about work or family matters. Stay aware of the joy of the walk and pay attention to where you are at that moment. Personally I find it more joyful to go walking on my own so that I can be alone with nature. Find some way to make your walk a special time for you, either with someone or on your own. Please remember this book is written for you and the sole purpose of it is to give you the incentive to move toward your healthier life style and a joyful and happier you.

Finally this is all you need to remember regarding this principle.

EAT LESS and MOVE MORE

The Big Lesson for Us All is:
To Learn to
RESPECT OUR BODIES MORE
– and Treat
Them At Least As Well
As Most of Us Treat Our Cars

CHAPTER ELEVEN

GOLDEN PRINCIPLE NUMBER FOUR

NUTRITION

Nutrition for me is one of the most enjoyable and thrilling subjects to read or write about. I love listening to others talking about this subject, discussing it with them, and giving talks about it, studying new developments and discoveries on the Internet or in books. Having said all of that however, I ask you to read the following pages of this chapter with a truly open mind, a sensitive heart and a sense of humour. I trust this will help you to make sense of what I wish to put across. However, if you don't agree with something that I write, may I ask you one small favour?

Don't say: 'No!' Just say: 'Oh!'

I feel that a real understanding of the true philosophy of nutrition is greatly lacking at present among members of the worldwide scientific community. It is not possible to appreciate the complexity of the nature and role of various hypotheses on nutrition when such things are viewed, as they still are scientifically, only from the point of view of facts, figures and materialistic forms of proof.

I know this is a very strong statement for me to make since large numbers of genuinely committed and decent scientists are diligently devoting a major part of their lives to seeking new discoveries. They also research constantly to find new ways to cure or eliminate disease. Yet as long as their scientific view is based solely on figures and materialistic proof, as far as human beings are concerned there will always be a different story to consider. You see human beings, rather inconveniently for science, are the only species on our planet that have choice.

Millions of years of evolution have led us to this present moment. Our main tool on this journey has been the power of 'focussed intention' or

131

the power of the human mind. However, this mind power has also thrown up some of the greatest obstacles to our achieving optimum health. One typical example is the way in which mankind has overcome many survival problems, including how to manipulate nature. Yet as a result we have forfeited a lot of our own natural instincts and our sensitivity to the Earth all around us.

For instance, we know every detail about all kinds of animals, from how much they eat, to how they sleep, their habits and natural habitats and what composes their nutritional diet. Yet we still fail really to know ourselves. Most of us are unable to recognise the difference between thirst and hunger in our own bodies, or to know what plant or food to use when we are not feeling well. Yet almost all other kinds of animals are in complete control of knowing what they need for their own wellbeing. This includes domestic animals. Try feeding a cat or a dog that is not well! My own observation and understanding is that in most cases they heal themselves by **RESTING** and **FASTING.**

In my humble opinion I think humans are the only species on Planet Earth who are confused in their understanding of their nutritional needs. There is no other animal that has this problem except us. One possibility could be that we go outside our nutritional boundaries and animals do not. It could well be possible, that this is why we are the only species that has false teeth.

Let me ask you a question or two: have you ever seen a lion, for example, sitting down and peeling an orange because oranges have vitamin C and are therefore good for him? Or have you ever seen a monkey, say, sitting down with a dish of fish and chips and while eating this food, washing it down with a so-called 'diet' soft drink? Or indeed have you seen any animal at all eating a nice slice of chocolate cake as a dessert with a strong cup of coffee? No of course we haven't seen any such things. We don't see them because animals eat only what they are supposed to eat.

You may ask me now: 'Well what are we naturally supposed to eat?'

Do you want to know my true answer? It is this: I do not honestly know beyond any shadow of doubt because over thousands of years of mixed-up eating patterns our instinct for the right type of foods has been lost.

Another cause of our confusion may come from the fact that there are so many theories and different schools of thought about nutrition and foods. Sadly some of these are contradictory to each other. I sincerely hope that I am not starting another one.

Before I go any further I wish to recall that Hippocrates, the father of modern medicine and the source of the Hippocratic oath which all modern Western doctors respect, used to teach his students to restore the unwell to health **FIRST THROUGH FOOD** and then through medicine. I do not know how or why but the majority of modern physicians seem to have lost sight of this simple and obvious fact.

Now, having said that, if you promise me that you won't jump out of your seat in frenzy at my impertinence, I will tell you what I personally believe we need for survival. Are you ready? You are sure? Okay, well here it is!

I believe that we can actually survive on four foods only! And they are: **QUINOA, DATES, GRAPES, and GARLIC,** further than that our body needs only one drink, Pure, Clean, and Clear Water. With these five substances in my opinion, all of our bodily food needs can be satisfied. And here are my basic reasons for adding these foods to our current diet.

- **QUINOA** provides vitamins, amino acid and protein.
- **GRAPES** provide all kinds of sugars and energy and cleanse our body.
- **DATES** provide minerals iron and trace elements.
- **GARLIC** is the best antibiotic, known for centuries, protects against infections.
- **WATER** a solvent that purifies the body. Remember: Water is life!

Because we are flooded by so many foods, particularly in Western societies, I feel the least we can do for our bodies is to add the above substances to our daily eating plan and if possible reduce a lot of other undesirable foods.

I believe I know what you are thinking at this moment. You want to ask me: 'Abbas would you like us all to go back into the cave with you, too?'

Well, not exactly. But what I want to tell you very simply is this: being healthy is not really complicated. Deep down we all know what is truly good for us and what is not. So are we just trying to fool ourselves?

Are scientists publishing their latest findings to support our current approach to food? No disrespect to scientists in general, but most medical scientific research funds are provided by commercial companies and they therefore have a vested interest in whether or not they allow publication of the research results. The main reason why they fund such research is to produce a food product or medicine that brings profit to their company.

So far there is nothing particularly wrong with that. But sometimes I feel things have gone a bit too far off of the rails. A comedian who was hosting the annual Hollywood Film Oscar Awards once said very tellingly; 'If there was a fire here right now and we all died, nobody could be identified, since everybody's teeth are made almost the same shape, same size or even have been fixed by the same dentist!'

There is a lot of unconscious truth in that joke because like those film stars in the Oscars audience, you and I buy similar services and products and we pay a lot of money for them: liposuction, face-lifts, breast enhancement, to name just a few in one area, are all available to us. The reason why these and other techniques are developing and becoming commonly available is because we 'buy into them'. We buy into the idea that they are necessary and valuable, whether that is really the case or not.

Here is another example I came across recently which is worth quoting.

Apparently there are scientists working at present on the genetic engineering of human blood to determine what kinds of disease a person might be susceptible to in the latter part of their life. The idea is that at birth you can give a few drops of blood that they can genetically modify to prevent the person concerned developing that disease in their old age. Sorry, this seems to be too late for you and me! We cannot become a baby again in this lifetime. But there are hopes for babies of the future.

Meantime, returning to our main subject, the truth is we would like to eat and drink everything and anything we want and to have no side effects at all as a result. Well I am afraid that is not possible. Everything has a price and we each pay the price of how we treat our body. In addition we now have so much choice that we are confused. If we could find contentment within a simpler life, that would be so much better!

I clearly remember how I used to suffer with headaches in my twenties. My level of wellbeing then was very low. Today I am twenty-two years older and I am very happy with my level of wellbeing. Yet when we get older we are supposed to be weaker. This is not the case with me and it does not have to be the case with you either or indeed with anyone who follows the wellness principles outlined in this book

Often when I am giving public talks on health, people make remarks about the clarity and brightness of my skin and particularly ladies make comments about how they would love to have that kind of fresh skin. So I tell them what I do and what I eat – and this is the response I usually receive: 'Oh, but I can't do that!'

So I ask: 'Why not? Everybody can drink two litres of water or so each day. We can do it – but we won't or don't do it. Therefore we end up with unhealthy skin, unhealthy hair and a generally ill body.'

So the big lesson for us all is:

**TO LEARN HOW TO RESPECT OUR BODIES MORE –
AND TO TREAT THEM AT LEAST AS WELL AS MOST OF US
TREAT OUR CARS.**

Would you agree?

Let's move on now and I will give you a small explanation about each of the four food items mentioned and I trust that perhaps you might then agree with me how important those foods are. I will deal with them in the order mentioned above.

QUINOA

The name of this food is pronounced **keen-wa** and it is a very nutritious 'mother grain' that was famously favoured by the ancient Incas of South

America. The Incas regarded it as one of their most sacred foods because it was so nourishing, delicious and vital and that is why they called it *chesiya mama* or 'the mother grain'. Quinoa is high in protein, calcium, iron, fat and oil, with a good balance of amino acids. Often described as 'a seed not a grain', it is gluten free and comes as close as any food to supplying all life-sustaining nutrients. Like Soya beans it is extra high in lysine, and is a good complement with vegetables, which are often low in methionine and cystine, both of which are amino acids. Also it is relatively good in phosphorous, vitamin E, and several of the B vitamins. It contains an almost perfect balance of all eight essential amino acids needed for tissue development in humans. Quinoa is 12% to 18% protein and four ounces a day or about half a cup, will provide and satisfy our protein needs for one day.

As already indicated it is not a true cereal grain but belongs to the chenopod group of plants – exactly the same family as the weed commonly known as *lamb's quarters*. It is said that those who try Quinoa for the first time characteristically respond by saying enthusiastically: 'Hey, this tastes good!' In fact I believe Quinoa is so good nutritionally that its impact gets through directly to the body with the message: 'Yes, this stuff is really good…I want more'.

GRAPES

Grapes are one food that can give you almost anything and everything that your body needs– most importantly energy. The flesh of the grape is a warm and wet food and the seeds of the grape are a cold and dry food. This combination makes grapes one of the most complete foods that exist. In addition the skins of grapes contain a well-known antioxidant called Resveratrol.

So grapes are in fact one of the best blood purifiers and also I like to call grapes **'BLOOD TRANSFUSION FOOD'** by this I mean that eating grapes helps our bodies to promote the production of blood and is available to all of us in such abundance almost all through the year, thanks to modern agriculture.

The sugar in grapes is a slow-releasing sugar and can enter the blood gradually to provide a great energy source. Grapes can improve the circulation and are excellent for the heart, chest and the urinary system.

If you want to lose weight you can eat grapes for breakfast and have nothing until lunchtime. But if you consume them with food or at other times you will actually put on weight. Grapes are known to be one of the best diuretics – this is why they are the best blood purifier and provide excellent tools to get rid of toxins from the body.

Eating about half a kilogram of grapes in the morning is a very good energy food after having a late night or if you feel tired in your head. What I am saying is that they are great medicine for hangovers! And almost all Persian writers have unanimously agreed that grapes are one of the best foods for prevention of cancer!

But let me end here with one small WARNING: Please do not consume cold water after eating grapes, as you may experience severe abdominal pain. My understanding for this is that the sugar of the grapes converts the pH of the stomach to high alkaline levels and consequently to heat, therefore drinking cold water is causing contractions to the stomach muscles.

DATES

Dates are an excellent and simple nutritional food containing all kinds of minerals and iron. Every 100 grams of dates provide more than three times the daily recommended dose of iron intake.

The best environment for growing dates is close to water where there is a lot of extreme heat and sunshine. Typically this will be by a riverside in a hot country. To flourish, all fruits need the presence of the four elements, **Earth, Air, Water and Fire or Heat** from direct sunlight. Dates require more than most – extra sun and extra water. That is why dates are as potent an energy provider as the **Sun** and as nourishing nutritionally as **Water.**

It is amazing that there is not much written in English health literature about these miracle foods. Eating dates with yoghurt is an excellent nutritional dish in any season, since dates are a warm and dry food and yoghurt is a cold and wet food. Both are on the lowest rank of the hot and cold food groups. That is why you can enjoy them at any time of the year.

If you like something that is a mild laxative in the morning, then you can soak about six dates overnight in a glass of warm water or any type of warm milk such as cow's milk, goat's milk, Soya or rice milk and then eat them for breakfast. Overall, please note: dates are a great all-round nutrition food.

Note: you may notice I mentioned a few times cold food, warm food, wet food and dry food. In Persia we categorise foods in these four groups and often we try to treat ourselves by adjusting some of our eating in order to overcome a variety of conditions, which is also grouped as cold or warm disorders. Please watch out for my next book which is going to be about '*foods to suit our personalities*'.

GARLIC

I think if you read any health literature at all, you will find that only good things are written about this excellent antibacterial and antiseptic herb. I remember being very impressed when I first read how 780 different pathologies of the human body can be relieved by the use of garlic alone. This was in a German study, I believe, released around 1990.

So Garlic is one of our very best natural antibiotics. That is why I put it on my list of daily foods in order to keep free from infections. It is at its most effective if you use it for six days a week and take a break for one day so that your immune system does not get too used to it.

Garlic can be taken via capsules or tablets. Also if it is grown organically it is very good. Nowadays most of the garlic supplements are organic but the most important thing to consider is how they process it without damaging the active ingredient of garlic which is called **ALLICIN**. Research indicates that garlic supplementation lowers the bad cholesterol and improves the ratio between **HDL** and **LDL** ('LOW' or 'HIGH DENSITY LIPOPROTEIN').

Garlic is among the group of plants known as **ADAPTOGENIC HERBS**. In simple terms this means that the herb adjusts itself to our body's requirements. An adaptogenic substance in formal terms is one that demonstrates a non-specific enhancement of the body's ability to resist a stressor. The term was first introduced in 1947 by Russian scientist N.V. Lazarev to describe the unique action of a material claimed to increase the non-specific resistance of an organism to an adverse influence. Then in 1958, a Russian holistic medical doctor, I.I. Brekhman, and his colleague I.V. Dardymov, established the following definition of an adaptogen: 'It must be innocuous and must not cause minimal disorders in the physiological functions of an organism. It must have a non-specific action, and it usually has a normalizing action irrespective of the direction of the pathological state.'

Some other examples of adaptogenic herbs are: red ginseng, called Chinese, Korean, or Japanese ginseng, white American ginseng, Siberian ginseng, Liquorice root and Astragalus are among others.

I trust that this brief summary of the benefits of these four foods will be helpful in encouraging you to make better and more balanced decisions regarding your own general health and wellbeing. Perhaps overall I feel that the widespread inability to understand the whole subject of Nutrition generally is not due to lack of knowledge but rather from too much of it. Also this knowledge is far too often contradictory. So let me try further to simplify.

* * * * * * * * * *

KEEPING IT SIMPLE
For the past fifteen years or more, I have thought that being vegetarian and eating wholesome food is the perfect health choice that we need to make – and eating too many dairy or animal products could cause a lot of health problems. But to my surprise I recently realised that this is not true in all circumstances.

Consider the following exception for example: I am sure most of us have either heard or read that the consumption of large amounts of animal food is the main cause of heart disease, cancer and diabetes. Yet now we see that shepherds in Kenya from different tribes consume half a gallon of milk daily and those who can afford it consume between two to four pounds of meat each day. They drink very little water, yet not only do they not have any of the above mentioned diseases; they are also among the fastest runners in the world with healthy arteries, fit bodies and strong hearts.

Why is this? How can it be? Well it is basically because they burn away what they consume. Therefore the consumption of large amounts of meat and dairy products does not affect them. Now you are going to say to me: 'Abbas, you are confusing me now. I used to think that there were Good Fats and Bad Fats! But now I am really confused.'

Well you don't have to be confused. Just look at our movement in Western life in comparison to people of those African tribes. If you eat heavy fat content food you must burn it up, otherwise your body has no way of using it as energy and it becomes overloaded, therefore health issues arise. The tribes we spoke of walk and run many miles per day, they burn what they eat with movement.

You can read more about this in the book by **UFFE RAVNSKOV MD** called '**THE CHOLESTEROL MYTHS**' then most issues of fat and cholesterol will become clear for you.

All you need to know is that if you follow the four simple, practical and do-able Golden Fundamental Principles of this book and apply them carefully, you will see open before you the heavenly doors of the healthy life you want. You might never have imagined that those doors even existed before – but they do and the key to opening them and finding your own special experience of health and wellness is only one small decision away. For some people the space between that decision and action is only one step. But for many that space is as wide as a large ocean that one struggles to swim across every day to get to the other side.

And that leads me to tell you another reason why I wrote this book. It was because, in spite of studying hundreds of health books I still felt confused. More accurately I can say I studied thousands of health books as well as health articles in magazines and scientific nutritional protocols. Yet the more I studied and learned, the more confused I felt, since most often one finding contradicts another. Now finally I have reached the stage that a Persian poet once described like this: MY KNOWLEDGE HAS REACHED THE POINT WHERE I FEEL I KNOW NOTHING.

So now after studying and treating people for years, I realise that the simpler the principle is, the more workable and do-able it will become. So that is another reason why you have this book in front of you at this moment! I want to make sure that what I have learned about the simplicity of **HEALTH AND WELLNESS** is being received by my patients, and as many others as possible so they may pass it on to others too.

I have found that in all of my years of experience working with people brought me to this conclusion: **It is not the power of the words that makes the difference in our lives, but rather the receptivity of the audience.**

Once I came across this quotation which I feel is strongly relevant at this point.

"THE STRONGEST HUMAN INSTINCT IS TO IMPART INFORMATION – AND THE SECOND STRONGEST IS TO RESIST IT"

What my desire is in writing this book, (and will later be on a larger scale with the 'Wellness Homes' mentioned at the beginning of this book, which it is my dream to set up) is to bring your attention to **Health** rather than to **Disease**. To encourage you to strive to find the *cause of your symptoms* rather than to just remove them, to encourage you never to be satisfied with a patched-up job concerning your health.

The underlying causes of **heart** disease and **cancer** are not specifically known or perhaps it's truer to say there are almost always multiple causes. They are the two biggest killers of our time, according to medical scientists, yet every year large amounts of public wealth is spent on research and investigation into the disease and very little attention is given to the prevention of these diseases.

Why is this the case?

Because medical scientists focus on the problems and try to find a medicine to overcome those problems, they usually look at it from a single and isolated viewpoint.

My wish would be that disease was looked at from a prevention point of

141

view and then the possibility of disease occurring in the first place would be lessened...

I notice that when I study a disease, I find I could spend my entire life on it, without coming to any end result. Millions are being spent on the study of disease and the end result usually has the comment '**The finding is inconclusive**'. Why is this? Could it be that we are looking in the wrong direction? I think the answer to this has to be, yes we are. The time and money could be used in a more productive way through health education and disease prevention. The way we chase disease at the moment reminds me of a scene of dogs chasing cars, have you ever seen a dog chasing a car? Most often they can't catch one and even if they could they would not know what to do with it.

In simple terms this means a lot of money and time investigating diseases has been wasted, and we still have no definite result. As I have already mentioned, over 150 pathologies are known to be caused by calcium deficiency. So wouldn't it be wise if we spent money on something simpler – like providing patients with supplies of absorbable calcium rather than spending millions of pounds on finding out how the disease is progressing?

* * * * * * * * * *

For the first time in a little while let me relate to you a story which will perhaps help explain more clearly some of the points I am endeavouring to make in this very important chapter. Perhaps we can call this story:

KEEPING THINGS SIMPLE IN PERSIA

A Persian friend of mine, who is a top medical consultant, was talking to me at a Persian party. He said to me: 'Do you know I was really ill with a cold for a few days recently. No matter how many antibiotics I used, they did not clear the cold.'

'So what did you do?' I asked him.

'Well one afternoon I was feeling so dreadful that I dragged myself home with the intention of going straight to bed. And my mother who was there at the time asked me: "What is wrong with you?" I told her I was not feeling at all well and she said: "Don't worry let me make some Persian style onion soup for you."'

I smiled at this and nodded. 'I think I know what's coming.'

'Maybe you do,' said my friend. 'Anyway after half an hour the soup was ready, and I ate two or three bowls of it before going to sleep for a few hours. When I woke up I was feeling much better. That night I was on duty, so I went to the hospital and I was okay. The following day I was totally better.'

'That doesn't surprise me at all,' I said. 'What did you conclude from that experience?'

'Well, I found it strange that there I was, having studied medicine for many years unable to clear my cold, and my wise mother with a simple Persian onion soup quickly cured my problem!'

Later on I heard that someone had asked my Doctor friend for health advice and he told him to go to Abbas to stay well and go to him with an illness. That may sound like a strange thing to say, but his point was this: doctors generally are not trained in health and wellness. Their training is mostly concentrated on diagnoses of disease and prescriptions of the right medicine for a particular pathology. Therefore they are not trained to give adequate nutritional advice or look at the root cause of diseases and identify them.

Hypothetically, even if they do find out or already know about a particular pathology, it isn't sufficient for them to just advise you of their findings. For example if a doctor finds out that the root cause of indigestion from which you are suffering, is that you are eating a lot of bread and jam, he can't just tell you to eat less bread and jam and send you home. If a doctor does that, after a while it might be thought that he is not a good doctor and does not go into things deeply enough. Or it may be suspected that you have a more serious underlying problem that was missed and not talked about. Therefore if something should subsequently happen to you, your family may sue that doctor for negligence.

Nevertheless, the right advice has to come from the right source. No one expects a plumber to understand electrical faults. That is the job of an electrician. Nor do you expect an urologist to give you advice about your heart. Often a doctor will clarify things for us by saying: 'This is not my speciality.'

Strangely, we seldom go to our medical doctors for health advice. If you don't believe me go to your doctor and say to him: 'Doctor I am feeling very well at present, can you give me some advice as to how I can stay well?'

What do you think your doctor would say to you? 'Well done! Go home and keep doing what you are doing. When you are unwell come back to me.' This is because the focus is on illness, whereas teaching people how to stay well will be an integral part of the Wellness Homes; the whole idea of them is to educate people on health so they can be responsible for staying healthy. More suggestions on Wellness Homes will follow our final golden principle on nutrition.

Now, let us continue with food and nutrition.

'COLD' AND 'WARM' FOODS

Here I wish to mention and explain in more detail something about 'warm' and 'cold' foods that I have touched on in previous pages. Also I would like say something briefly about other forms of the healing arts that are derived from different cultures.

In Chinese medicine for instance, practitioners focus on cleansing the body by stimulating the liver and then balancing a person's constitution by opening their meridian points and releasing energy blockages. Then they will give adequate amounts of herbs, tincture, or other ingredients of Chinese medicine in order to maintain and balance that wellbeing. In Ayurvedic Medicine – Ayurvedic means 'life knowledge' in ancient Sanskrit – they divide people into different body type groups. The information for each group type will determine which kinds of food a person needs to have and what kinds of food to avoid, no matter what the pathology or symptoms or disease.

The ancient Persian Healers known as Hakims worked around the

Golden Principle Number Four

principle of Food Unity which is a term I am just using here to express something of the basic Persian healing wisdom and its methods and treatments for maintaining wellbeing in different stages of health – as well as for restoring health from the conditions of disease. I have not come across any Western writing about this subject in terms of dividing food and diseases into 'cold' and 'warm' categories – with the exception of books on Food Combining and Blood Type Diets. But even these writings do not give full significance to knowledge that exists about foods which fight in the stomach or foods that are complementary to each other.

By the way when I say 'warm' and 'cold' foods as I have done a few times in preceding pages, I do not mean their *temperature* but rather each food's basic nature. For example melon is categorised among 'warm' foods and both tea and coffee are categorised amongst 'cold' foods, which terms are contradictory to their usual temperature when we eat and drink them in the most common way. Also in the Western diet, drinking orange or grapefruit juices with breakfast cereals containing milk is very common, yet this combination can cause major digestive problems. Let me explain why, simply, citrus juices taken with milk causes the milk to go sour in the stomach which can be the cause of indigestion disorder.

There is an almost endless list of this kind of information of course, and I will now give you a brief taste of it, so to speak. The first person in Persia who started to match pathology with 'cold' and 'warm' foods was **Mohammad Ibn Zakariya al-Razi** who lived in the ninth century A.D. He was popularly known to the world as Razy or Al-Razi and you will find more biographical details about him at the end of this book.

Razy worked by determining the underlying cause of a disease from the colour of the patient's skin at the moment of the illness. He then would change the medicine as the colour of the skin changed. Today we understand this from the types of secretions of bile from the liver to the gallbladder. Bile enables us either to digest or not digest food, and one thousand years ago this man not only knew this, he even practiced it. Today this kind of approach would be laughed at by modern medicine, yet the unanswered question in my mind is this: in spite of the great advances in medicine and in spite of spending large amounts of wealth on healthcare services, why do we still end up with our hospitals filled to capacity? A high percentage of the people in hospitals are suffering from chronic diseases, which are rapidly rising. *So we must be doing something wrong!*

In today's healthcare service, everything is transformed into academic terms and even patients' heads are full of academic information. Also, most importantly, we are being fed the idea that more is better. We are encouraged to feed more, take more drugs, have more operations and in fact have more and more of everything. For my part the only 'more' I feel that I can agree with is: **MOVE MORE.**

THE OPERATION WAS SUCCESSFUL – BUT THE PATIENT DIED

I have been thinking for months or even years now about the same question connected with what I have written above. It pops into my head all the time and it is this: 'Where exactly are we going wrong?'

Put another way the straight question might be framed as: 'What are the core problems of our health services today and how can we do more to prevent illness?' Well after a great deal of thought, I am setting out here the way I see things.

As long as the conventional medical community is not being educated in the most fundamental area affecting our health, which is **NUTRITION** and is not prepared to listen then nothing will change. I have heard that medical students at their universities spend no more than a few weeks studying nutrition during the whole of their seven years and this fact speaks for itself. The outcome of this neglect will be that our health will get worse and worse as time goes by. Sadly not only does the conventional medical community not seem to wish to listen to people like myself on this subject, they are sadly very often dismissive of the whole subject. Yet they are sitting in the seat of authority as far as the public's health is concerned.

Nothing will change in my view unless you and I demand health services which bring greater standards of health and wellbeing instead of continuing on a course of action which is clearly on a wrong track – even though it appears to work with high levels of precision.

Incidentally, I trust I am not giving you the impression that I am disrespectful or unmindful of the amount of knowledge that medical science has given us. Nothing could be further from the truth. Everything about our human body that we know today is a product of the painstaking efforts of thousands of medical scientists and nobody should underestimate this. But my point is this: Are we getting healthier as time goes by – or are we becoming unhealthier?

What good is the following statement which I placed at the head of this section and which I have truly sometimes heard?

The operation was successful, but the patient died.

The whole purpose of the operation is to make the patient well. If the patient is not well then the operation was a failure, no matter what level of precision has been achieved. I know you are going to say: 'But Abbas, we know all of this. Why are you telling us again? There is nothing new in this.'

That is the sad part. Have we become so used to such statements and circumstances that we think we cannot do anything about them? Do we really feel we have to accept whatever conditions we are served up?

I feel any medical practitioner or alternative physician must honour their position. We trust them and put our lives in the hands of physicians, especially and naturally when we are ill. All of us can feel vulnerable, sometimes we even feel mentally and emotionally weak. We need to realise that medicine can only offer certain things. But also a lot can come from the level of understanding and trust and the interpersonal chemistry that needs to be established between patient and physician.

Personally when I look back on cases of my own that have been successful, I see that my patient and I felt that we understood each other and that we knew what to expect from each other during the healing process. Believe me the correct or incorrect medicine had very little to do with it! In fact this chemistry was the same in all the cases that either were successful or not.

FOOD UNITY

Let us continue now by talking further about FOOD UNITY, which is common knowledge among Persian people. It is almost like a common language. For example there are quite a few well known tenets and here are just some of them:

- Do not eat jam while you have a cold or flu.
- Always eat at least one orange after eating nuts and seeds.
- Do not mix citrus fruit with liquid dairy products.
- Do not eat many cold or many warm foods together.
- And most importantly eat foods that are 'opposite' to the season. For example cold foods in warm seasons and warm foods in cold seasons.
- And in the springtime have cleansing foods.
- In autumn eat mild and gently warming foods.

All of the above mentioned points are effectively **Persian Health Proverbs** and have a connection with people who suffer from certain kinds of pathologies which I have seen in people in the Western world, as a result of not applying the food unity principles. There is an abundance of writings regarding 'cold' and 'warm' foods in Chinese medicine, Indian medicine, and also both ancient and modern Persian medicine in original Persian writings. But as I said earlier I have not seen or heard of this style of treatment in Western medicine either alternative or orthodox.

I personally had a lot of encouraging results using this knowledge when I was operating in my health food store. I would spend only a minute or two giving suggestions to people to add a certain food at a particular time when they were experiencing a particular pathology. Most of that knowledge I just remembered from the daily advice given to me by my granny.

For example for a person who has a cold sore, I recommend to eat broad beans two or three times a week. Not only will the symptoms subside a great deal within a week or two but in some cases they never actually return. When the person concerned changes his or her diet and adds broad beans to dishes regularly, the missing piece of the puzzle called **NUTRITION DEFICIENCY** is found and replaced.

Did you know that cold sores are the lack of an essential amino acid called **LYSINE** and broad beans have lots of it? So you can see that a problem can be approached from the source and then the cause will be removed. Once this has been done, usually those same problems do not return. You can take **ANTIBIOTICS** as long as you like but you will never solve a problem that is caused by a nutrition deficiency

When I was in Persia, I did not know why we ate certain foods in particular circumstances and I had no access to textbooks to find out why we did this. Now anyone can keep up to date on nutritional needs particularly with the advance of the Internet. Today we have access to a vast amount of information.

Most of the advice at home just went from generation to generation without being recorded anywhere. Here in the Western world, however, very few physicians seem to follow the root purpose of these suggestions. But it is important to add to that the fact that here in the Western world I personally have learned more about **ANATOMY, PHYSIOLOGY AND PATHOLOGY** and have consequently married the two strands – Eastern wisdom with Western modern medicine – and that appears to have given me an overall picture of health.

This is another area which I promised myself I would write about sometime in my life, so that I could share with you how, in Persia, illness is treated first with food then with herbs and medicine. Prescription of medicines would be only a temporary measure and after health was restored the prescribed medicine would gradually be discontinued under the advice of a competent physician. I am sure that in most countries many ancient healers had this very simple wise way of healing illness.

Somewhere we have lost the essence of healing in our modern medicine, we need to look at the way we use pharmaceutical medicine and how we have become a society which has become dependent on medication, looking for a quick fix from illness. Please don't get me wrong, I know medicine has a place and plays a major role in saving lives every day, but not in the way we have become dependant on it. Our focus on illness has just made us unhealthier and we are reaching major crises, and are being forced to look at other ways.

To become a well society we must focus on **Wellness not Illness**.

I say this because I speak about **HEALTH** and **WELLNESS** not only from an academic point of view, otherwise this book would be just a theory nothing more. I have studied and applied the wellness principle to large numbers of people and obtained great encouraging results; this is why I am writing about the information and knowledge behind it all.

That is why I am repeating over and over and over in these pages about the importance of seeing things simply. You can read this book for pleasure or study it very intently or just read one page at a time. Or if you are as lazy as I am you can just read the highlights of the four Fundamental Golden Principles and apply them regularly and you will win big time in your life.

Yet as we all know, not everything which is **SIMPLE** is **EASY** to do. It does take discipline and resolution and other qualities like persistence and awareness.

But before I go any further I feel another story coming on and I would like to tell it to you. It is called:

THE STORY OF A MISCHIEVOUS MAN WHO WAS SEEKING A CITY TO LIVE IN

Once upon a time there was a mischievous man trying to find a city where he could live comfortably and not have to do much. On his travels he was accompanied by a donkey and a hen, which he owned. One afternoon he arrived at a farm and asked the farmer if he could please tell him of a short cut to the nearby city?

The farmer replied: 'Why do you want to go to the city?'

'I am running out of money and I need to find some work,' the man replied. 'And as you can see I have some animals with me that I need to feed.'

Golden Principle Number Four

'Why do you travel with those animals?' asked the farmer.

'Well the Donkey is cheap to run and the Hen lays an egg every day,' replied the man. 'So one gives me free transport and the other feeds me. So I have an easier journey with them. But I am always open to suggestions.'

After thinking for a moment the farmer asked him 'How much money do you have?'

The travelling man mentioned an amount of money which was very little in Persian currency.

'Then go that way,' the farmer told him, pointing out a direction. 'About one mile from here, you will arrive at a fruit and vegetable stall before you reach the city. With the amount of money you have, you can buy a large melon, eat the melon yourself and that would satisfy your thirst and hunger. Give the skin of the melon to the donkey, and the seeds of the melon to the hen. Remember the melon will satisfy your hunger and thirst and also give you energy to continue your travelling for another day. Who knows by tomorrow God will possibly bring another blessing in your life.'

The travelling man thanked the farmer and continued his journey. But to the farmer's surprise, the man began to walk in the opposite direction to what he had suggested.

The farmer called after him, asking; 'Why are you going that way? That is the opposite road that I suggested to you.'

'My friend,' called the travelling man in reply. 'In a city where the local farmers are that smart and still have to work hard for a living, I will have a very hard time finding suitable work. So I am on my way to somewhere else.'

This story has been circulating in Persia for centuries about a city called **HAMADAN** and this name literally means ALL KNOWLEDGEABLE and people of that city and all intellectual people in general are famous for such qualities.

The reason I use this story here is because of its **NUTRITIONAL** content.

As is mentioned in the story the nutritional value of the melon for three different (human and animal species) digestive tracts is a good tool for me to get across the following points I wish to make:

FIRST POINT: Experiments carried out on animals with either foods or medicines cannot be one hundred per cent reliable for humans. Also not all foods and medicines which are safe for animals are safe for humans.

SECOND POINT: We need to consume foods the same way as all animals do, that is to say foods, which are suitable for our biological activity. Also we need to remember that foods, which are not suitable for us, can cause many disorders and diseases.

I very strongly request that you PLEASE carefully ponder these two points. Really sit with them for as long as you can, until you have a clear picture about them. They are vitally important to understand and absorb.

Here I wish to share with you two very extraordinary facts about the direct connections between nutrition, health and illness. An Australian doctor has a slogan which goes like this:

EIGHTY PER CENT OF ALL DISEASES ARE OUR OWN FAULT!!! ONLY TWENTY PER CENT ARE BAD LUCK.

By 'bad luck' he meant hereditary. Second, did you know that **Almost all deaths except accidents are caused by nutrition deficiency, no matter what age the person is!** Yes, these really are true statements that the majority of nutritional experts are only just coming to terms with.

I quote these two startling facts because I can't otherwise begin to tell you how important nutrition awareness is in determining the level of your health. Neglect this knowledge and you are likely to pay a heavy penalty sooner or later. I do promise you that if you knew and understood fully the value and magnitude of good daily nutritional habits you would not even waste one minute before implementing them. But I will do my best to pass on to you as much information as possible without boring you.

Golden Principle Number Four

This chapter, I repeat, is about **NUTRITION** the last of the **Four Golden Principles of Health and Wellness**. But although it comes last it should not be considered any less important than the other three. In fact all four principles have the same equal value and I find the best way to remember them is to imagine each of the four principles as a separate wing of a steadily spinning ceiling fan. To be truly effective each blade of the ceiling fan must play an equal part in stirring and circulating the air. So it is with the four principles. That is why I see them as four equally active arms spinning horizontally at an even rate rather than principles that move up and down (see Diagram 3, page 48).

When we apply just one of the principles fully in our life that will give us about twenty five per cent of the overall maximum credit that the four principles together can pass to our general Health and Wellness 'bank account'. Therefore applying the fourth **NUTRITION** principle can do the same for us and give us twenty five per cent of the overall benefit. In fact I see the four separate 25 per cent contributions adding up to one hundred per cent as representing the amount of effort that we need make if we are truly to get the level of health that we wish for. So to make sure there is no misunderstandings about this I confirm the obvious – that the twenty-five per cent effort, which is required for each of the four principles does, if applied correctly, bring about one hundred per cent optimal health and wellness. So now let's look even closer.

To be most effective the **Fourth Golden Principle 'Nutrition'** must be divided into two separate portions that are quite distinct from each other. They are as follows:

- **PORTION ONE:** A proper nutritional diet with fresh foods, preferably organically grown in our own environment, requires twenty per cent of the total effort to bring about the level of **HEALTH AND WELLNESS** that we desire.

- **PORTION TWO:** Five per cent of our total effort needs to be allocated to the consumption of naturally grown **ORGANIC SUPPLEMENTS**. I really believe this! I mean, how much time would it take to swallow a few organically grown food supplements every day?

These are such important distinctions that I will deal consecutively with the Two Portions in detail and spell out what is required to make the practice of them both most successful.

FOURTH PRINCIPLE – PORTION ONE:
A PROPER NUTRITIONAL DIET

There is not a day goes by without our hearing about some new report or article on the importance of eating sensibly. By now you may have noticed that I am using the term **EATING SENSIBLY** instead of **EATING HEALTHILY**.

In my many years of experience with treating and counselling people about their health, I have come to feel that the expression **EATING HEALTHILY** cannot be universally agreed or applied and cannot be considered an objective statement since one food can be so helpful to someone's health, yet the very same food can be like poison to others. You will perhaps remember my earlier story about the barber and the tailor in ancient Persia and how one became well with beans and cider vinegar and the other died.

So I prefer to use the expression **EATING SENSIBLY** and by that I mean we should generally eat and drink in such a way so as not to belabour or overload our body. If we are suffering from any illness, as we regain our health with the help of competent physicians, then we can choose to gradually widen our range of health promoting foods and drinks in order to sustain health and wellbeing.

ALLERGIES

To elaborate on the statement I made above about different foods being suitable or unsuitable for different people, I'd like to give you this example: fruit and vegetables are universally considered to be good nutritious foods. Yet they can be poison to a person who suffers from a stomach ulcer. Or take another example, such as grapes. Generally grapes are the most wonderful fruit one can imagine from a nutritional point of view. Yet they can be the main cause of chronic diarrhoea for a person who suffers from **DIVERTICULITIS** or **DIVERTICULOSIS** or indeed any form of colon disorder that prevents them from enjoying the benefits of this heavenly fruit. To give yet another similar example, some

Golden Principle Number Four

people who appear to be healthy generally with no symptoms at all, have a severe allergic reaction to nuts.

Please note that the following advice is aimed at those who suffer from normal to moderate allergies and I would advise all people who suffer severe allergic reactions to consult with their health practitioner.

Here are my own clinical experience and suggestions on the subject. In general terms I would say that if you have any form of allergy regarding any type of food or drink you can consider doing as follows: take small amounts of the substance on a regular basis, then gradually build up to an adequate quantity until you are able to have normal amounts.

For example if you are allergic to wheat or milk, just take a grain of wheat or a drop of milk every day for two weeks. Then gradually increase the quantity of that substance to which you are trying to overcome your sensitivity. This is a well-established method by means of which you can gently promote the production of particular digestive enzymes in your system.

Now you may wish to ask: What if my allergy is to grass or paint? Well my answer to this is: first of all do not eat them! I trust you will excuse my humour here! I just wished to ensure that there was no misunderstanding!

Becoming serious again, from my experience I have come to realise that the majority of allergic reactions come from a person's immune system being weak. So by boosting the immune system almost all kinds of allergies can be overcome. Please note I said 'almost all kind of allergies'. There are some cases, I have found, where the underlying cause is very obscure and needs months or even years to get to the root of the problem. Also please note carefully that the ability to tolerate certain foods and the speed of overcoming food sensitivities can vary greatly from one person to another.

There are many more examples I could give you to illustrate this. For instance, as far as drinking more water is concerned, some people find it very difficult to accustom themselves quickly to the higher daily amounts that are essential for true wellness. It may take at least six to twelve weeks for their bodies to adjust to the new fluid balance that results from the introduction of larger quantities.

Anyway, I will not bore you with further examples because I trust that by now you have got my point.

FOURTH PRINCIPLE: PORTION TWO: SUPPLEMENTS

It took me almost twelve years of seeing with my own eyes the good effects of consuming organically grown supplements before I was convinced that they were absolutely essential for the lifestyle which we live today.

My thinking used to be this: if we eat well we can overcome all health issues. But I was wrong. The overwhelming evidence of scientific facts forced me to accept the need of supplements in our daily diet in order to reach our optimal health target.

One internationally known Australian cardiologist said this about the use of carefully chosen supplements:

Paying for supplements is like paying pension contributions – you receive the benefits from them in the long run.

So we also need to look at this situation in the same way that we look at paying for our health insurance – which is very different from our present circumstances, where we have to pay for our recovery from illness. If the medical industry treated humans the same as animals we would be better off, because most animals receive regular nutritional supplements as part of their routine diet and we humans don't.

I heard from a doctor who worked as a zoo animal vet, who said: 'If we treated animals like humans our burger would cost $298 dollars. And if we treated humans the same as we treat animals the insurance premium for a family of four would be two dollars and fifty cents per annum.'

It seems to me that the zoo vet has a very good point!

Also there is plenty of scientific evidence to prove that the use of supplements is more effective over the long term than if used short term or in 'start and stop' patterns. It is quite certain that taking supplements

Golden Principle Number Four

can prevent the development of many diseases like heart disease, cancer, diabetes and many others.

When we talk about supplements we of course come to the subject of vitamins. The word vitamin was first coined in 1912 by an American biochemist named Casimir Funk, after he discovered the disease beriberi, which developed as a result of the lack of B vitamins. The word vitamin was an abbreviation of the two words VITAL AMINES, the essential amino acids needed by all living cells. Then after some time the two words were joined and the AL and E were dropped.

Sometimes we find out something that becomes very obvious once we have discovered it– yet the truth about it has often previously seemed so different. One example is that we all now know that the Earth is round. But there was a time when it was not common knowledge.

In this connection I remember very clearly the night that I escaped from Iran to Pakistan through the desert of Sistan and Baluchestan. On that night we had to stop in the middle of the desert and there the scenery was breathtakingly beautiful. But I was so nervous that we might be caught that I could not enjoy it during our break from driving.

When I think back to those moments, I feel I was like a tiny ant in the middle of a clay dish with a blue lid on. It was very hard to believe then that the Earth is round and the sky is only endless space. No matter how much Galileo might have tried to convince me of those facts on that night, it would have been extremely hard to understand his point. Today of course this is elementary knowledge. Everybody knows that the Earth is a round planet. But there was a time when no one believed Galileo and his theory.

I wonder if it is possible that the way we think and what we believe about health today will be very different in another hundred years. I firmly believe it will be.

And might the day come when we actually believe and know that neither medicine nor the physician can bring about a cure? The truth is that the cure can only come from within. Could it be that as in the time of the 'flat earth' theory before Galileo we are so convinced by our current understanding of everything in our surroundings that we won't allow any space for new ideas?

The answer to that question in my view is of course: Yes! But why should this be so? Is it because new ways of thinking and understanding will shake our old ideas or beliefs and therefore make us feel unsafe? Again of course I suggest the answer is: Yes!

Let me give you an example to explain my point: Only a hundred years ago scientists thought that there were things in fresh food that caused illnesses– like viruses in fruit and vegetables. But today their thinking is different. We now know the things that we miss if we don't eat fruit and vegetables, like the lack of vitamin C, can be the cause of diseases like scurvy and the lack of B vitamins can be the cause of beriberi.

Furthermore, in recent years researchers have found links between people who suffer from arthritis – osteoarthritis or rheumatoid arthritis – and the lack of a trace element call Boron in their body.

The total amount of boron in the human body is about three grams. That is somewhere near the equivalent size of a few poppy seeds. Yet the lack of it can be the cause of one of the major autoimmune deficiency illnesses. Can you see the miracle of creation within the human body when a tiny amount of trace elements, can have such an effect over disease. This is why I wonder whether the lack of other vitamins and minerals could be the cause of the ever growing number of diseases which mankind is suffering from.

I remember when I started taking supplements, I could not get myself disciplined enough to use them according to the manufacturers' recommendations. A month's supply of a multi-vitamin and multi-minerals would last me for a few months. But now my wife Carmel and I arrange for a company to deliver our monthly supply of supplements on a standing order basis, this way we do not need to remember every month to purchase them, and over time we have created the good habit of taking them daily. This not only saves us time but helps in keeping us at our optimal health.

So my suggestion to you at this point is, make one decision like this and follow it – even if you do not see any results for a few months. Believe me it is quite certain that in the long run you will reap some considerable benefits.

DIFFERENT SUPPLEMENTS HELP MALES AND FEMALES

It has become clear that the constitution and metabolism of the male and female bodies are different and that they benefit from taking slightly different supplements. So I would like to suggest some different ranges of **VITAMINS, MINERALS** and **HERBAL MEDICINE** for males and females.

Please consult with your physicians – whether they are from the conventional medical sphere or the complementary sector – about applying these suggestions in your daily diet. Ensure you do this, particularly if you are on prescribed medication.

As well as showing these different medical advisers respect, it is important for them to know what is happening with the progress of your health and it can then be better monitored.

For both sexes the use of multi-vitamins and multi-minerals with some trace elements are highly recommended; and wherever possible purchase organically grown food supplements. There is a considerable difference between synthetic supplements and natural food source supplements of which you should be aware.

- **SYNTHETIC SUPPLEMENTS** isolate a specific vitamin or minerals.

- **NATURAL FOOD SUPPLEMENTS** are made from concentrate or extract from various fruits, vegetables, or plants, which contain **PHYTO NUTRIENTS.**

Please be warned about the words **NATURAL SOURCE.** Some manufacturers use this term yet in spite of this, the process and production of their supplements are **SYNTHETIC**. Legally they are not breaking the law since the source of their products is nature. For example all petroleum-based ingredients and those that come from the seabed or ground rock are all called 'natural source' since they come from nature.

One of the most disturbing and misleading forms of labelling occurs when the words **MINERAL OIL** are used. This usually means **PARAFFIN**, which is added to raisins and sultanas in order to prevent them from sticking together.

Another label warning to watch out for are the words **NO ARTIFICIAL SUGAR ADDED**. This usually means the product has ordinary sugar. It is simple to check it out, because if this is the case, it will say somewhere on the label that the product is not suitable for diabetics. There are many other labelling tricks used so it is good to scrutinise the labels carefully. For now I hope that some of this information will be of help to you in choosing the most suitable products. In general I will just say:

ALWAYS INSIST ON BUYING ONLY ORGANICALLY GROWN FOOD SUPPLEMENTS

Now let me give you some specific guidance on the different supplements that are specifically helpful to males and females. Reversing the gentlemanly principle of 'Ladies First' just this once, I will begin by describing what is good for my own gender!

FOOD SUPPLEMENTS ESPECIALLY GOOD FOR MALES

First I would like to recommend an herbal medicine called **SAW PALMETTO** with the added ingredients of **PUMPKIN SEED OIL** and **NETTLE ROOT EXTRACTS**. I do this because a high percentage of males over age fifty are dying from prostate cancer and a large number of these deaths can be prevented.

One of the main problems with prostate cancer amongst men is that it takes between four to ten years in order to develop, and even though they do have urination sensations at night for that period of time, most men do not attend a proper physician until it is too late to do anything about it.

SAW PALMETTO or *serenoa repens* has long been used among Native Americans. In some medical communities it is a well accepted herbal medicine with no side effects. So if you are a male aged 40 or over you could find great benefits in taking this magic herbal medicine sooner than later.

I am over 50 years old and I take it. I also take other supplements like

Golden Principle Number Four

MULTI CAROTENE and **BILBERRY.** These two products are great for prevention of degenerative eye disorders; I take them because I read study and basically use my eyes a lot. If you are happy with your eyesight then you do not need to use them but you may choose to include them in your diet to guard against complications with your eyes.

Nowadays there is a lot of talk about **FREE RADICALS** and the advantages of using **ANTI OXIDANTS** for prevention of major diseases. We largely live in an environment where it is impossible to avoid absorbing large amounts of free radicals into our systems. Among the sources are **AIR POLLUTION, PASSIVE SMOKING, FOOD ADDITIVES** and **STRESS.** Therefore taking a good multi-vitamin multi-mineral supplement with antioxidants is an important move to consider.

The source producing free radicals that is the most dangerous and which we need to do everything possible to avoid, I would say is **STRESS.** This is the only free radical source that we have control over. One famous survey has shown that a high percentage of heart attacks among men take place on a Monday morning, as we are all preparing to return to work after a weekend off. So I wonder why that should be!

Having said that let us now turn to the much beloved fairer sex and discuss what supplements are good for them.

FOOD SUPPLEMENTS ESPECIALLY GOOD FOR FEMALES

First and foremost I would recommend for the ladies the regular use of **EVENING PRIMROSE OIL** or **EPO.** And by 'ladies' I mean every female from the age of fifteen upwards to any age. But let me sound a firm **WARNING NOTE** here: Please do not use **EPO** if you are on epileptic medicine.

Some manufacturers have cleverly combined **EPO** with other ingredients like **BORAGE SEED OIL** also known as **STARFLOWER OIL, GINGER EXTRACT, DONG QUAI,** and **CHASTEBERRY** also known as **AGNUS CASTUS**

All of the above mentioned herbal supplements have for centuries proved to be beneficial to the wellbeing of women in every part of the world.

Also I would like to suggest the occasional use of **CALCIUM** and **MAGNESIUM** supplements, preferably the chewable variety because that way they digest better. It is good to wash them down with orange juice because orange juice accelerates the absorption of the so-called '**Cal-Mag**' into the blood stream. The greatest beneficial effects from **Cal-Mag** are likely to be felt by women who are already aged forty or over, women who suffer with PMS or PMT – pre-menstrual syndrome or pre-menstrual tension – and women who have weak bone structures. But this particular supplement, it must be said, is very good indeed for the wellbeing of all women in general.

Again, as with **EPO** above, there is a clear **WARNING NOTE** to be sounded here. The use of **Cal-Mag** almost always brings about a sensation of wellbeing in women who take it, yet it is not advisable to use **Cal-Mag** permanently. You can vary the duration from three months to two years but you should always give your system a break by taking the supplements via a pattern of six months **ON** and one month **OFF**. When taking **Cal-Mag** for the first time it is recommended to stay on it for at least 3 months to feel its benefit, since it takes sixty to one hundred days for cells to regenerate.

Some women are pleased to find that taking a herb called **BLACK COHASH** is also very beneficial for the balance of hormones, and mental and emotional harmony. There are also many other supplements and herbal medicines which can contribute significantly to a woman's health and wellness but to discuss these fully and give accurate advice it is necessary to have more details about each individual's constitution, age, diet and other factors. But all the above mentioned supplements are in common use by women all around the world.

SUPPLEMENTS BENEFICIAL FOR EVERYBODY
Now to end this section of the Fourth Golden Principle I would like to broaden out the subject to discuss a further group of supplements that are beneficial for both males and females. Some of these are already well known and a few not so well known. I will start by looking at oil.

FISH OIL
In recent years the use of supplements composed of fish and fish oil has

become very widespread and popular in the western world. Particular credit should be given to an essential amino acid called **OMEGA 3** that has already been well documented. Considerable research has already been done and more research is still being carried out on this product. The benefits it brings include improved lubrication and use of our joints, improvement in the sharpness of memory and general improvements to the wellbeing of our heart and circulation.

CLA

CLA stands for conjugated linoleic acid and it is a close relative of linoleic acid which is the essential fatty acid found in sunflower oil and other vegetable oils. It was 'discovered' nearly twenty years ago and its properties are still being researched intensively at universities around the world. Among other things it is believed that CLA can help our body's immune function and perhaps reduce body fat and promote lean muscle mass. It is obviously an important chemical and I write more about its discovery and potential further on in this chapter under the subject heading of **OBESITY**.

VITAMIN E

Vitamin E has lots to offer us in the realm of health benefits. Most importantly it helps improve the general wellbeing of the heart and circulation, improves the elasticity of the skin and helps counteract dryness of the skin, particularly in women and so has a positive effect on the early appearance of fine lines or wrinkles in the face. It is also one of the best known **ANTIOXIDANTS**.

VITAMIN C

It is widely understood that our daily need for Vitamin C is as great as our need for daily bread. However agreement on the strength of the daily use of this supplement varies widely from one school of thought to another. Nevertheless my understanding is that since this is a water-soluble vitamin then we can never overdose on it – providing, I would add, that its source is an organically grown food source.

The need for vitamin C in our daily diet is almost as important as our need for air and water. The most important benefits obtained from it include: prevention of immune disorders; protection against hayfever and its reappearance; prevention of chronic diarrhoea; assistance in cell reproduction; prevention of all kinds of infections and finally it is also, like Vitamin E, one of the best known anti oxidants.

VITAMIN B

There are many types of B Vitamins each one serves different needs. When you use Vitamin B it is much better to purchase a B-complex package which contains all the B Vitamins together. Nowadays most of them also have folic acid included. B Vitamins are very important for the health of the central nervous system.

They also improve the balance of fat in the blood, can prevent colon disorders as well as generally aid the wellbeing of the digestion tract.

There are many other vitamins, minerals and trace elements which are important for our well being. Amongst them are **CHROMIUM, SELENIUM, BORON, MOLYBDENUM, ZINC** and many others. Also in recent years herbal supplements have became very popular. Herbs like **GINKGO BILOBA, ECHINACEA, CRANBERRY, LIQUORICE** and **GINSENG** have their own special great benefits to bestow on us. Some are very good for boosting our energy, some bring about general improvements in our wellbeing and most of them have been used for centuries. The subject is worth studying in greater detail than I have space for here; it is in my view an urgent matter that you consider immediately beginning to add at least some of these supplements to your daily diet based on the outline I have given. So to round off this section on the Fourth Golden Principle I would like to introduce the following quotation to help give further urgency to your decision:

AN ERROR DOES NOT BECOME A MISTAKE UNLESS WE FAIL TO CORRECT IT.

SOME GENERAL POINTS ABOUT NUTRITION

It is worth saying here that **EATING SENSIBLY** or **HEALTHILY** in fact is not hard at all. It is really only a matter of taking the time to change a few small habits, nothing more! A high percentage of people who are health conscious today were not always that way. Something triggered them to change their eating habits

The majority of health conscious people start to eat sensibly because either they become ill and are advised to change their diet or they notice their own appearance is changing and this makes them think more seriously about their health. Unfortunately a lot of people only change to more sensible ways of eating after they get some kind of alarming health warning. But it doesn't have to be that way. You can start eating sensibly now, straight away after reading this book! By choosing to expand your knowledge before you became unwell! This is like:

DIGGING A WELL BEFORE BEING THIRSTY.

To elaborate on these few essential general points about good nutrition, the majority of people easily tolerate fruits and vegetables. So eating adequate amounts of them, either steam cooked or raw, is one of the best health actions anybody can consider taking.

Also we need to remember that food preparation is very important. For instance **POTATOES** are best eaten when they are cooked in their 'jackets' or skins. It is in this form that they give us their highest nutritional benefits. The next thing, however, that we often do with the potato is to make chips or French fries from it. In this form we not only lose some nutrition we also add fat and free radicals into the mixture. The last and worst thing that we do is to make the potato into crisps. Now this really is the time when we lose all the potato's best nutritional value and exchange it for unhealthy – or even to some degree harmful – food. At all stages the raw material is the same – the **POTATO**. The only question is: how do we prepare and cook it to gain the best nutrition from it?

There is lots of information about the benefits to be gained from eating fruits and vegetables. You can even find out about which of them is most effective for the prevention of particular illnesses or conditions. It is very good to educate yourself in the habits of eating that are best for you, so I am not going to say much more on this. Instead I would like to share with you some of the latest information on nutrition that can be taken advantage of right now even though, as far as I know, it is not yet widely known to the general public because the data is still in its rawest form.

Excuse Me! Is This Your Body?

The story goes like this: imagine **YELLOW LEMONS, GREEN PEPPERS** and **RED TOMATOES** lying side by side in your kitchen or on your dining table. All of them contain vitamin C but scientific research is now discovering that the effects on the human body of the vitamin C from a yellow lemon are different to the effects of vitamin C from a red tomato or a green pepper. Yes, you have guessed it – colour counts and nowadays food scientists are putting the focus of their research very much on the colour of fruits and vegetables and some plants and flowers like Marigolds which are not suitable for human consumption. But it is now known that these plants, fruits and vegetables contain types of phyto nutrients called **LUTEIN** which is beneficial in the prevention of many kinds of eye problems.

The other connected discovery that is now becoming well established is that communication between cells in fruit and vegetables takes place via their colours.

Apparently there are over 600 **PHYTO NUTRIENTS** in fruits and vegetables. But less than 100 of them have been named and isolated so far. Some research has been done on them but the remaining 500 are not yet fully understood and their efficacy has not yet been fully established.

So based on this new information, my suggestion is this: every time you make salads of either fruits or vegetables, please remember to put in them all the lovely rich colours, **RED, GREEN, YELLOW, ORANGE** and **BLUE.** You can use berries for the blueness or even blue cabbage. Do this even if the ingredients are from the same family. For example use small amounts of all the different coloured peppers instead of just one colour. On this subject I love the following quote from a famous Persian doctor who wrote several books on the advantages of eating fruits and vegetables daily. He said:

IF THERE WAS A SHOP WHERE YOU COULD BUY AND SELL HEALTH, I AM SURE THAT WOULD BE A FRUIT AND VEGETABLE SHOP.

He also is famous for asking his patients a certain question as he watched them swallowing unpleasant medicine for advanced illnesses about which they had no real choice:

WOULD IT HAVE BEEN EASIER IN THE FIRST PLACE TO HAVE EATEN THE DELICIOUS FRUITS AND VEGETABLES?

He does have a point, doesn't he?

Now let's look briefly at that modern health scourge that is undermining the wellbeing of increasing numbers of people, particularly children, in Western society – obesity.

OBESITY

In recent years a great deal of research has been conducted into the condition of obesity – particularly obesity in children, which in the United States and some parts of Europe has become very widespread. Because of this and also because obesity can seemingly be the source of many other illnesses, it has become a major target of investigation.

However; my understanding of obesity is this: Like all other chronic diseases **OBESITY** is not a single, simple, symptom, it is a combination of complex disorders, which have **PHYSICAL, MENTAL** and **EMOTIONAL** causes. But if we are going to confine ourselves to one clue or one area that we need to look at more closely, I will of course suggest **NUTRITION**.

Apparently there is a great deal of agreement amongst all food scientists that obesity is a symptom of malnutrition and by feeding the body proper nutrition a lot of issues around obesity can be overcome. I try to look at solutions rather than problems; therefore I am saying it here again. Focusing on obesity is like focusing on the problems. Yet if we can see the source of the cause and remove it, hopefully obesity will soon not be as big an issue as it is today.

By focusing on three of our four Golden Principles – **EAT LESS MOVE MORE, WATER** and **NUTRITION** – a lot of health problems can be overcome, including the issue of obesity.

I hope you will truly see the power of these four Golden Principles and not take them for granted. They are the synthesis and essence of hundreds of theories, studies and personal experiences so a lot of detailed knowledge lies behind these seemingly simple and workable principles.

Excuse Me! Is This Your Body?

Some time ago a new discovery was made as to why we as a planetary race are seemingly **BECOMING EASILY OBESE**. As always I will keep it as simple as possible so here is just some of the theory.

Many people assume that being overweight is a failure of self-control. But that isn't exactly true. There are many more forces at work, including the vast changes we have made during the last century in agriculture and lifestyle that affect how our body responds to food. Now, at last, science is beginning to understand more of the mechanisms involved and we can begin to streamline our body to better effect.

One of the discoveries that may help us in our efforts to do this comes from an unexpected source. Back in 1978 Michael Pariza, a scientist, was investigating the chemicals that form when burgers are cooked on a charcoal grill. The concern at that time was that mutagenic or cancer-promoting amines might be formed during the grilling process. But Pariza unexpectedly found something in the burgers that had quite the opposite effect. It took him ten years to isolate and identify this chemical from beef, which eventually turned out to be a close relative of linoleic acid, the essential fatty acid found in sunflower and other vegetable oils. Pariza called his discovery conjugated linoleic acid, or CLA.

CLA has, in the event, turned out to have some very interesting properties and is increasingly being researched at universities around the world. For example, studies to date suggest that CLA can benefit the body's immune function, cardiovascular health, blood sugar management and bone health. But perhaps most interesting of all to those who are oversized, is that CLA appears to act as a partitioning agent, a nutrient that reduces body fat and promotes lean muscle mass.

One of the questions that scientists and the overweight want answered is: why do people get overweight so much more easily today than they did twenty years ago? One answer may be that there is now a lot less CLA in our diet. CLA occurs naturally in beef and dairy fats, including cheese and whole milk. But cattle only get their CLA by converting some of the linoleic acid they get from their traditional food – grass. In recent years cattle have been fed grains and other feeds instead and there is now a lot less CLA in the average human diet.

WHAT IS PARTITIONING FAT?

As athletes know, the body is made of two major types of tissue: body fat and lean body mass. Everyone knows where the fat is – around the girth, hips, thighs, and upper arms in particular. The lean body mass makes up everything else, muscles, organs and bones. Athletes are constantly striving to increase or maintain lean muscle mass and reduce their body fat. And that is what every oversized person should be trying to do as well. Just dieting to lose fat is unwise, because you are likely to lose muscle mass as well. And when you gain weight again, as you almost certainly will, it will be fat that you gain for the most part, not muscle. This raises an important viewpoint, which we need to correct if we are to reach our goal. We want to be slimmer and fitter, and we think that the way to do this is to lose weight. So we hop on the scales every morning and develop an obsession with the verdict at our feet. But when we look at other people it isn't their weight we're looking at, it's their shape.

When we fixate on the scales we forget that it's our shape we really care about. Weight is just a shorthand way of checking our progress, not necessarily an end in itself. But does this matter? Yes, it does, for an important reason. Lean body mass is heavier than fat.

So the first sensible step to take in moving ourselves towards a better shape and weight is in short to: burn fat and build muscle. Every dieter dreads the flabby loose skin people can develop when they lose weight. What they really want is a lithe, toned, well-developed body. The way to achieve that slimmer and fitter shape is to reduce body fat while maintaining or developing lean muscle mass, and since lean muscle is heavier than fat, we could end up with a thinner, more streamlined body without a particularly big change on the scales.

The first clinical study involving CLA took place in 1997. The purpose of the test was unknown to the people involved and some ten volunteers were given just over a gram of CLA at breakfast, lunch and dinner, and another ten people were given placebo capsules. After three months the average body fat of the CLA group had dropped by twenty per cent, whereas the body fat of the group that took placebo capsules was unchanged. The CLA group had also lost about five pounds in weight, although there had been no change to their diet and nor had they been asked to exercise.

There is evidence too that CLA can help gain muscle size and strength following exercise. A group of twenty-four novice body builders took 7.2 grams of CLA a day or placebo capsules while on a six-week body building training course. The CLA group had greater gains in arm size and improved by about seventy pounds in the strength test. The placebo capsule group made only half these gains.

The precise mechanism behind these effects is not yet fully known. Scientists suspect that CLA helps to mobilise fat out of fat cells and decrease fat uptake into those cells while enhancing the body's ability to burn fat for energy in the muscle tissue. Over time this decreased fat cell uptake and enhanced muscle metabolism will help decrease the size of fat cells in the body, while enhancing muscle mass. As fat decreases and muscle mass increases, the result is a leaner, trimmer and healthier body. "CLA makes fat cells release fat into the blood," researcher Michael Pariza explains. "The skeletal muscle can then burn the fat." Combining CLA with continuous aerobic exercise for 20-30 minutes and 2 plus litres of water per day is the best way to quickly burn up these free fatty acids circulating in the bloodstream.

I am trusting that this section in particular and the whole of this eleventh chapter on the Fourth Golden Principle is giving you a great deal of food for thought. I trust too that you will find it all useful and informative and will manage to put the information and insights into practice in your life.

Finally to conclude the chapter, I am going to tell you this brief short story, perhaps best entitled:

THE FRUITS OF HEAVEN
When I was in the military, a friend asked me in front of a group of

Golden Principle Number Four

soldiers this question: 'Is the olive one of the Fruits of Heaven?'

I responded without any hesitation: 'Yes'.

'Why do you say that?' he asked.

Again without any pause I responded: 'Because in Heaven there are all kinds of fruit, including the olive.'

When I look back, I can see that there was more wisdom than I perhaps realised at the time in this reply of mine. And yes, all these years later it does seem even more certain to me that all fruits and vegetables will be and are available in heaven. And it also might be true to say that if you would like to end up in heaven later rather than sooner, you'd be better eating, whenever you can, all the different kinds of fruits and vegetables that already exist so deliciously abundant for us here on Earth.

And please most of all remember that this book was written for **you**. It is for **you**, and the sole purpose of it is to give **you** the incentive to move towards a healthier lifestyle and to create as quickly as possible a joyful and happier **you!** So to do that, you need to keep this vital principle in mind always: **Eat less and Move More!**

* * * * * * *

I would like now to briefly share two **WELLNESS HOME** suggestions which could be introduced in order to change the present healthcare circumstances and create healthier lifestyles.

1 Establishment of health and wellness home via a **GOVERNMENT BODY.**

2 Establishment of health and wellness home via the **PRIVATE SECTOR** or **NGOs** (NGO is a Non-Government Organisation).

I personally feel if the Government would take this idea on it would be much more in alignment with the development of our society, nevertheless the idea of convincing any government about something as revolutionary as the **'WELLNESS HOME'** and have them act upon it, seems like a big challenge to me.

Perhaps if someone were to privately start a Wellness Home and make it a success then maybe government organisations can copy them and make Wellness Homes more widely available for everybody.

But either way can be just fine, as long as we start doing something. I am sure as I explain, it will be clearer and easier to understand.

In my first suggestion, I would like to propose that governments apply the wellness principle to one or two nursing homes. Why nursing homes? Because people who live in nursing homes have very little mobility and often they are on medication. And most importantly they can be monitored as often as the health programmer wishes, and they can be observed and evaluated based on a 24 hours monitoring programme. So when progress is achieved within this kind of environment, then the application of the wellness programme in younger generations and people with no needs of regular medications would become more promising.

Please note this kind of work has been done before, but with one difference: the purpose of the work was to prove a particular theory and after it finished the programme was discontinued. My point is this, in a Wellness Home, not only would we learn how to change the way we treat illness, but also learn to focus on wellness, use less medication, and give a better quality of life.

Another thing governments can do is to apply the four principles of this book to hospitals, which would have no adverse effect on anybody. In fact governments can do a lot. For example most hospitals are looking for more room to house ill patients. The focus on this adds to and prolongs inadequate health care systems. When the focus is on wellness a lot of the space which is now overcrowded by ill patients would be freed up. This could be then used in more productive ways, by putting in place a policy where every hospital would have a dance room, exercise room, swimming pools, story telling rooms, laughing rooms, and…rooms…rooms…rooms… where healing can take place. Can you imagine the effects of those activities and how much improvement can be brought about in the lives of patients? It is blowing my mind why such simple and effective laws of wellbeing became so complicated, and nothing is being done about them.

Golden Principle Number Four

I hope I am making sense to you. In reality the principle of wellness can be as wide as we wish, and as creative as we like, since human minds are the unbounded territory. So there is no limit to how many good things we can do.

As you can see I can keep on going with many more suggestions which could make this book a very heavy one. I would not be surprised if you told me more effective and workable suggestions yourself, and I would welcome them very much. But for now we will leave it like this.

So let's talk about running it in a private form. Basically what I mean by privately running a Wellness Home is similar to that of a commercially run business, where someone takes the idea and offers the services of wellness and wellbeing as a business venture. Many private companies are in business because of the service they give to people who are unwell, so why not have a business which offers wellness and wellbeing instead.

I have total and absolute realisation of the complexity of my suggestions, I know it needs to be planned properly and have lots of committed and devoted individuals to bring about those plans. I personally have a plan for the private sector and if you are one who has an interest in this venture and wish to pursue this project further, please feel free to contact me and maybe we can do something great together.

In my humble opinion, I feel the most needed ingredient to bring the Wellness Home or Wellness Programmes to fruition is the **'PASSION FOR HEALTH'**. Everything else is a secondary requirement, but passion is the first and the most important one. The passion I have for bringing this project about is what gives me the energy to make my dream a reality and see **WELLNESS HOMES** come into existence.

We Are All Just Like
A Single Cell
In This Body We Call
HUMANITY

CHAPTER TWELVE

HEART TO HEART

In this last chapter my desire is to talk from my heart to yours. May the words in the next few pages reach your heart in a conclusive way and may you feel their lightness like the lightness of a butterfly, flying freely from my heart and landing gently on yours. I hope at least that by this time you can feel some tingling sensations!

In writing in the Introduction to this book about the picture on its cover showing our heart as the Financial Control Centre and Treasure Chest of all our organs, I also said that our heart is not just an organ but rather it is the centre of our whole being. Also while our heart is obviously in our body, we are also paradoxically in our heart too. **Your Heart is in You and You are in Your Heart,** I said, and I added: The only reason you will apply the information in this book in your life is, if it makes you feel good in your heart. You may have an idea of whether that has happened by this stage – but in case you are still wavering, I would like to express one last time the wish for it to touch your heart enough for you to take action on your own behalf and take full control of your own wellness – and help others around you to do the same.

By now of course you will be expecting me to tell one last story – and I confirm that your expectation is to be fulfilled! Not too long ago an African boy told me this story and I would like very much to share it with you. The African boy started like this:

THE HEART OF GOD
'God', he said, 'created us in six days and on the seventh day was having a rest and thinking to himself: "Where shall I place myself so that I will always be close to them?"'

'Well God went on thinking for most of that day,' the African boy continued, 'and finally the answer came. He decided to place himself in our hearts. And why did he do that? Well this was the reason he gave:

175

'Your heart,' said **God** to us, 'is the place where I can be close to you always...When you are feeling joy or sorrow, in your success and in your failure, in times of fear and in times of faith, and especially when you feel **LOVE,** I will always be there with you.'

That was the story. It was very short and very simple. Yet it touched me so much because it reminded me that I am never alone. It reminded me that whenever I listen to the voice of my heart I can make a connection with my Creator.

The power in the words of this story can lift our hearts at any time. Its simplicity is its power. If you can grasp its simplicity, you will feel its power.

In this book I have shared with you some of my personal learning and experiences, which I hope will be of use to you in your life. I am well aware that there are still many things for me to learn and I look forward to growing and learning much more on this wonderful journey of life. They say the only room that exists that has a lot of empty space in it, is the room for improvement.

During our lifetimes we gather beliefs day-by-day that are opinions either learned or gained from others, that we then hold to be true. That is because *Homo sapiens* are the only species that has been given this gift of belief. This tool is the internal engine that has given us the energy to move forward up to the current moment of our human existence. Sadly sometimes this tool of belief is used in a negative way. For instance we can too often believe that our way is the only way and harm or kill others in trying to insist that they need to have the same beliefs as us. Sadly in many cases in our history, this way has led to destruction and war in which many people suffered.

On the other hand, much more often our belief can act like the small flame of a fire that keeps us warm. It is the only real hope we have to help us reach our goals and fulfil our dreams by doing things that are good, right and true. **BELIEF** is certainly one of our most powerful tools when it is used wisely.

Now, what I am hoping is that this book has brought to you a form of

BELIEF that can bring joy and happiness into your life just like the well known 'placebo effect' which is often observed in studies of how best to treat different illnesses. Most of us know that a placebo is a totally inactive or inert substance like sugar that is usually given to half of a controlled group of people who are taking part in a trial of some new medicine.

Although they have deliberately been given nothing effective to cure them they don't know this and they spontaneously acquire the **BELIEF** that what they are taking is going to heal their ailment. Consequently their condition often improves. I am not of course making an exact comparison or meaning to suggest that this book is in any way equal to an 'inert substance'. As you already know, it is my firm belief that it contains many truly effective and active measures we can take to improve our health. What I mean by comparing it to the placebo effect is that I hope that it will trigger a similar response in you based on **BELIEF**.

More and more pharmaceutical companies are resisting this 'placebo effect' discovery in every way possible because, there is a good chance that it will provide a new understanding to the public, which is that pharmaceutical drugs are not as necessary as we at present believe them to be. It is the same in different trials for headache, heart disease, or stomach ulcers despite the fact that the body needs to produce different chemicals to treat these different ailments. Yet it has been proven that the body can do what is required for its recovery just through the person believing they are taking a medicine that will cure them, when in fact they were only given an apparently useless placebo. As we know, such **DIS-EASES** can only be cured by secretions of totally different chemical activity in the body – so the only mechanism that could have brought about a cure for their illness was the **BELIEF** that the new drug they were taking was going to cure them. This is an amazing phenomenon and gives some indication of the mystery and power that is lying dormant within us. We have literally been given the gift of curing ourselves without outside help by **BELIEF** alone.

Also it is now known that when any discovery is made, that knowledge can quickly become universal by some mysterious means. The proof of this is provided by a scientific study or experiment that has come to be known as **The Hundredth Monkey Syndrome**. The explanation goes like this:

A group of scientists were studying the behaviour of monkeys on an island somewhere around Japan and they noticed that the monkeys there liked to dig up the roots of sweet potatoes or yams. The monkeys at first spent a lot of time brushing sand and dirt from the sweet potatoes before they ate them. Then the scientists observed at one point that one monkey was washing his yams in surf on the beach before eating them.

This was obviously a much more efficient way to clean the yams. Well, the scientists kept watching and watching and eventually there were two monkeys washing their yams in the sea, then four, then six, then eight and before long the scientists noticed that all the monkeys on the island were following suit and doing the same. But then something ever more extraordinary happened. The scientists found that the moment that all the monkeys on their island starting doing this, all the monkeys on other islands nearby started doing it too.

So it became clear that there was some sort of invisible connection between the animals and once a critical mass of one hundred monkeys became involved: **BOOM!** The behaviour and knowledge suddenly went totally subconscious and almost immediately all monkeys were doing the same.

Can you imagine? If monkeys have enough intelligence to receive a new discovery via universal signals or some strange sixth sense, then we as human beings must have it too.

Visualise this: by you deciding to implement in your life the Four Golden Principles for Wellbeing and Good Health outlined in this book, there is a strong possibility that it can spread to your family and friends and maybe to your community. Before we know what has happened there could be thousands of people like you following and acting on these principles.

Imagine it like this: there are thousands of candles and just one match.

The candles in themselves cannot ignite their own flame they need an outside source; the match also cannot light all the candles as it has a limited life time to burn. But if the match only lit one candle then the rest can be lit by each other.

My hope for the book is that maybe it can be seen like the match, and if one heart's flame is ignited to stir the passion for health and then passes it to others, many flames for a passion for health can be lit.

I am not the owner of the Four Golden Principles that lie at the heart of this book. I would like to think of its contents as a match. The Four Principles are all yours and what you do with them from now on is entirely up to you. If you decide to take their advice and become healthy, the joy it will bring to my heart will be immeasurable. The reason I say this, is because I know when you follow the principles the results of success are not only possible but inevitable.

Let's come back for a moment to this book and the **BELIEF** that I am hoping will be passed on to you. Let's just pretend for a moment that everything I have shared with you in this book has no value whatsoever. But since the information is not harmful in any way you decide to apply it in your life. This would mean that out of every three people who read this book, one would become well by just having the **BELIEF.** I hope what has been said in these pages will be truly helpful in your life for achieving **HEALTH** and **WELLNESS.** When this happens that will be the time I will feel my **GOAL** has been fulfilled.

But before we close this book let me tell you one last story. It is called A STORY OF AN ANCIENT SCHOLAR and I invite you to read it just for fun – and also take it with a pinch of salt! Oh! Or maybe not!

A STORY OF AN ANCIENT SCHOLAR
Once upon a time there was a great ancient scholar who wrote several books on various subjects concerning spiritual life, some of these works ran into many hundreds of pages and others into many volumes. For example he wrote many books on the meaning of the word 'Angel' and about such things as life after death; he also wrote of his ideas on the profound meaning of 'true human life'.

Apparently, one night he dreamt that he had died and was in line awaiting his turn to go through the gates of Judgment. While he was waiting in the queue he began to listen to the questions and answers that people gave to the Guardians of the gate. What he heard went something like this: **'What is it that you believe?'** People would say what their belief was and each time the Guardians of the Gate would look at the book of judgement and send them to the rightful place that they deserved. The scholar felt very confused. How is it possible to be this easy?

When it was his own turn he complained to the Guardians. 'Your procedure of judging appears to be too simple,' he said. 'You ought to be more thorough in examining different people and their understanding of spiritual knowledge.' One of the Guardians replied politely: 'We do not need your advice here, thank you; this is the time and place where we make the decisions.' After a short pause the Guardian asked: **'What is it that you believe?'** The scholar drew himself up to his full height and said: 'I believe in God who is beyond any form of description in words or objects or images and it is not possible to apply to Him any material meanings. He is the QUINTESSENCE of the QUINTESSENCE of the QUINTESSENCE of the TRUTH.'

The Guardians were stunned. The one who was holding the book looked at it open-mouthed and discovered he could find no such description. So the Guardians asked the scholar to please wait until they returned and, leaving him outside the Gate, they went to God and told Him about the strange gentleman. God listened patiently to their description of what the great scholar had said. When they had finished, He smiled quietly in response: 'Oh, don't be concerned,' he told the Guardians. 'I know him and his beliefs. He is perfectly okay. He is a very harmless man – let him go into heaven! And don't mind him or his descriptions about me. Because when he was alive on earth he wrote so many volumes of books about me that I can't even understand them myself...'

Just at that moment the scholar awoke with a start from his dream. He sat up abruptly in bed, staring wildly into the darkness. He was much shaken and he stayed sitting bolt upright for a very long time. For several days, despite his tendency to babble, he spoke to nobody at all. Then at last he began to recover from what had been a serious fright and from then on he became very easy going. He made it clear he was not in the least bothered about differences in people's beliefs and often he would talk and laugh about this dream with his friends and students.

Now how true this story really is I cannot say, only God really knows, I suppose. But every time I read a highly sophisticated scientific research analysis or read the law about property or a television programme on religious debates, I remember this story. I like and cherish it because I feel we take life so seriously most of the time, we need to chill out a bit.

If we could only follow and visualise this sentence: '**We are all just like a single cell in this body we call Humanity.**' We may find it difficult to sustain this marvellous visualisation – but if we could do it, then life would be much easier for everybody. Also the life of the world's rich and poor people would not be as it is today, where half of the amount of money spent on chocolate in some wealthy countries could feed all the people of another. Let's pray the day will arrive soon when the world will become a different place. Right now the people in one part of the world are ill because they eat too much and in another part of the world they are ill because they do not have enough to eat.

I look forward to the time within the next few months when I hope to receive letters or e-mails from you telling me how you have applied the Four Golden Principles of this book and achieved a great deal of wellness. Of course if you choose not to contact in the traditional fashion, please remember when you reach your desired goal of **HEALTH** and **WELLNESS** I will congratulate you from the bottom of my heart and will take great pleasure in celebrating your achievement with you in the realm of infinite possibility known as **THE QUANTUM FIELD.**

And now dear reader I take this opportunity to write one last time of the importance of the establishment of **HEALTH AND WELLNESS HOMES,** where the focus is on staying well and the use of food and natural remedies would be the first step in restoring health – and hopefully working alongside the medical profession in teaching and educating people on wellness principles. That is my dream!

And as I take my leave of you here, dear reader, please keep in mind this Old Persian proverb which says:

When you were born, you were crying and everybody around was smiling. So strive to become the one who, when you die, is smiling and everyone around is crying, because they will miss your presence in their life.

Finally I would like to leave you with a telling phrase that my teacher passed on to me many years ago. Even now I feel it to be a great blessing which serves perfectly as a last word for the main narrative of this book.

EVERY JOURNEY BEGINS WITH THE FIRST STEP.

So go on! Take that first step and start today. You've got nothing to lose. But you have a whole world of happiness and a joyful life to gain – and may God bless you on your way!

APPENDIX

GREAT NATURAL HEALERS

PAST AND PRESENT

Throughout this book, as you have already seen, I have combined wisdom ancient and modern in my efforts to present eternal truths about how we can best achieve good health and wellbeing. To conclude, I will just mention a few details about four outstanding men, two from ancient times and two from the present, who I am convinced deserve our acclaim and gratitude.

The 'ancients' are Ibn Sina, also known as Avicenna, and Razy – in full Abu Bakr Muhammad Ibn Zakariya Ar-razi whose Latin name was Rhazes. Both these outstandiong men lived over a thousand years ago. The 'moderns' are Dr Fereydoon Batmanghelidj, an Iranian-born, US-based doctor who sadly died at the age of 73 in November 2004, and Dr Patch Adams, an American doctor, who has been immortalised recently in a famous Hollywood movie. I will do my best to present and honour them chronologically.

Let us start with **Ibn Sina**, a Persian physician of long ago, who as indicated above, was perhaps best known as **Avicenna.** He was born in 980 AD at Bukhara in Iran and died in 1037 at Hamadan.

The most famous and influential of all the philosopher-scientists of Islam, Avicenna is particularly noted for his contributions in the fields of Aristotelian philosophy and medicine. He composed the **Kitab Alshefa – The Book of Healing**, a vast philosophical and scientific encyclopaedia, and the **Canon of Medicine**, which is among the most famous books in the history of medicine.

Avicenna was an ethnic Persian who spent his whole life in the eastern and central regions of Iran and received his earliest education in Bukhara under the direction of his father. Since the house of his father was a meeting place for learned men, from his earliest childhood Avicenna was able to profit from the company of the outstanding masters of his day. A precocious child with an exceptional memory that he retained throughout his life, he had memorised the entire Quran or Koran, the Muslim scriptures, and much Arabic poetry by the age of ten. Thereafter, he studied logic and metaphysics under teachers whom he soon outgrew and then spent the few years until he reached the age of 18 in his own self-education.

The Canon of Medicine (Qunon) is the most famous single book in the history of medicine in both East and West. It is a systematic encyclopaedia based for the most part on the achievements of Greek physicians of the Roman imperial age and on other Arabic works and, to a lesser extent, on his own experience although his own clinical notes were lost during his journeys.

In medicine the Canon became the medical authority for several centuries, and Avicenna enjoyed an undisputed place of honour equalled only by the early Greek physicians Hippocrates and Galen. In the East his dominating influence in medicine, philosophy, and theology has lasted over the ages and that influence is still alive within the circles of Islamic thought.

Occupied during the day with his duties at court as both physician and administrator, Avicenna spent almost every night with his students composing these and other works and taking part in general philosophical and scientific discussions related to them. These sessions were often combined with musical performances and gaiety and lasted until the late hours of the night. Even in hiding and in prison he continued to write. The great physical strength of Avicenna enabled him to carry out a program that would have been unimaginable for a person of a feebler constitution. So his masyery of health matters was truly reflected and confirmed in his own remarkable well-being.

The man best known to the world as **Razy** was born in roughly 865 AD at Ray in Persia (now Iran) and died somewhere between 923 and 932 in the same city. As already indicated his name in full was Abu Bakr Muhammad Ibn Zakariya Ar-razi and in Latin Rhazes. **Ar-razi, Razy or**

Rhazes was a celebrated alchemist and Muslim philosopher who was also considered to have been one of the greatest physicians of the Islamic world.

One tradition holds that Ar-Razi was already an alchemist before he gained his medical knowledge. After serving as chief physician in a Ray hospital, he held a similar position in Baghdad for some time. Like many intellectuals in his day, he lived at various small courts under the patronage of minor rulers. With references to his Greek predecessors, Ar-Razi viewed himself as the Islamic version of Socrates in philosophy and of Hippocrates in medicine.

Ar-Razi's left two significant medical works: the first is the **Kitab al-Mansuri**, which he composed for the Ray ruler Mansur ibn Isaac and which became well known in the West in Gerard of Cremona's 12th century Latin translation. The second is the **Kitab al-Hawi, The Comprehensive Book**, in which he surveyed Greek, Syrian, and early Arab medicine, as well as some Indian medical knowledge. Throughout his works he added his own considered judgment and his own medical experience as commentary. Among his numerous medical treatises is the famed **Treatise on the Small Pox and Measles**, which was translated into Latin, Byzantine Greek, and various modern languages.

These two outstanding physicians and sages have perhaps been little known popularly in the West in modern times and it is my modest hope that this book might in some small way begin to help change that and foster some interest in their great achievements and insights.

* * * * * * *

Moving on now to the present day, **YOU ARE NOT SICK YOU ARE THIRSTY** is perhaps the most famous identifying phrase associated with an outstanding modern Iranian, Dr. Fereydoon Batmanghelidj, who is the author of a worldwide modern health best-seller entitled **Your Body's Many Cries for Water,** which has sold more than a million copies worldwide. 'Dr. B' or 'Dr. Batman', as he is widely and affectionately known throughout the world did extensive research on the subject of water for almost 25 years.

Excuse Me! Is This Your Body?

He was born in Persia in 1931 studied medicine at St Mary's Hospital, London University and practiced in Tehran until 1979 when along with many other innocent middle class Iranians he was dragged into prison to be shot during the violent revolution that overthrew the Shah. While awaiting trail, he discovered the healing powers of plain water by prescribing a single glass for a prisoner dying of acute stomach pain. The man recovered – and Dr Batmanghelidg saved his own life by presenting a research paper on water to the presiding judge, who rescinded the death penalty and decreed a shorter sentence so he could expand his study of the subject.

On his release in 1982 Dr B escaped to the United States. There he helped set up The Foundation for the Simple in Medicine to explore and communicate his discovery that chronic unintentional dehydration is the true cause of many modern illnesses. He is also the author of related books entitled **How To Deal With Back Pain and Rheumatoid Joint Pain, Eradicate Asthma Now With Water, Water Cures, Drugs Kill, Water and Salt, Your Healers From Within** and **Obesity, Cancer And Depression – How Water Can Help Cure These Deadly Diseases.** Through these books and associated CDs, Video tapes and DVDs, Dr Batmanghelidj's work is gradually becoming more widely known every day and I am sure one day his revolutionary medical breakthrough will be widely recognised.

Dr Batmanghelidj stands out globally with **Dr Patch Adams** who is equally famous for his **Gesundheit** or **Laughing Clinics**. He is well known for saying IT IS TIME TO GET OUT OF THE BOX !

Dr. Patch Adams is certainly not one of the many people who are content to believe that the current health services are the best that there can be and that we can not change them. And thank God not all of us feel that way... There are thousands of physicians particularly in the medical community who do not believe this concept so they are trying to change it. Dr. Patch Adams and Dr Batman are among the leading pioneers in this field. Dr Patch brought a new idea to the world of illness and gave to people a new vision about how to get treatment for mental health via helping others; a book written on this subject, is entitled **The Secret of Living is Giving.**

Appendix

Dr. Patch Adams with his great mind and wonderful sense of humour, created the **GESUNDHEIT** or **LAUGHING CLINIC** which today is helping thousands of people around the world to overcome their particular mental and physical conditions.

You see Dr. Patch and Dr. Batmanghelidj decided not to stay in the box of **CONDITIONING**. And now as you reach the end of this short book, it is your turn to reflect on all you have read in these pages and decide for yourself:

Am I going to stay in the box ?

Or is it time for me to move on?

ACKNOWLEDGMENTS

I would like to thank a few very special people

First, my great friend Adel Shaphipoor has given me his constant support by providing many Persian resources and words of love and encouragement. I am particularly grateful for his prayers of support for the success of my work on such a scale that I am speechless as to how I could voice my appreciation.

A very special 'thank you' must also go to my very dear friends Anthony Grey in England and Ms. Maria Watkins in Ireland for the very substantial contributions they made in helping get this book into print.

Finally there have been many people from modern physicians to ancient Persians who inspired me greatly and I have used some of their material in this book. Among the many from my own country I have chosen only to write about three of them here in the foregoing Appendix but my gratitude to them all is boundless.

CONTACT INFORMATION

For anybody who wishes to make contact with me either about the concept and practicality of setting up Wellness Homes or any other aspect of this book, the contact details for telephone, e-mail, internet or postal letters given below should be used. I thank you most sincerely for taking the time to read this book. That is the only thing that makes writing it truly worthwhile.

     E-mail: ghadimia@gofree.indigo.ie

     Telephone: +353-56-7761525

     Postal: Fernhill, Dunningstown, Kilkenny, Ireland

     Internet: www.tagman-press.com